STUDY GUIDE TO ACCOMPANY
NASM's Essentials of Sports Performance Training

Brian Sutton, MA, PES, CES, NASM-CPT

Scott Lucett, MS, PES, CES, NASM-CPT

Editor

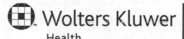
Wolters Kluwer | Lippincott Williams & Wilkins
Health

Philadelphia • Baltimore • New York • London
Buenos Aires • Hong Kong • Sydney • Tokyo

Acquisitions Editor: Emily Lupash
Product Manager: Andrea Klingler
Marketing Manager: Christen Murphy
Production Editor: John Larkin
Designer: Teresa Mallon
Compositor: Aptara Corporation

First Edition

Copyright © 2010 Lippincott Williams & Wilkins, a Wolters Kluwer business

351 West Camden Street   530 Walnut Street
Baltimore, MD 21201   Philadelphia, PA 19106

Printed in China

9 8 7 6 5 4 3 2 1

Library of Congress Cataloging-in-Publication Data

Clark, Michael A.
  Study guide to accompany NASM's essentials of sports performance training / Michael A. Clark, Scott C. Lucett, Brian G. Sutton.
      p. ; cm.
    ISBN 978-1-60547-912-5
  1. Physical education and training—Examinations—Study guides. 2. Sports medicine—Examinations—Study guides. I. Lucett, Scott. II. Sutton, Brian G. III. National Academy of Sports Medicine. IV. NASM's essentials of sports performance training. V. Title.
    [DNLM: 1. Sports Medicine—methods—Examination Questions. 2. Exercise—Examination Questions. 3. Exercise Movement Techniques—Examination Questions. 4. Physical Fitness—Examination Questions.   QT 18.2 C594s 2009]
    GV341.C556 2009
    613.71'1076—dc22

                                                                          2009012316

DISCLAIMER

Care has been taken to confirm the accuracy of the information present and to describe generally accepted practices. However, the authors, editors, and publisher are not responsible for errors or omissions or for any consequences from application of the information in this book and make no warranty, expressed or implied, with respect to the currency, completeness, or accuracy of the contents of the publication. Application of this information in a particular situation remains the professional responsibility of the practitioner; the clinical treatments described and recommended may not be considered absolute and universal recommendations.

The authors, editors, and publisher have exerted every effort to ensure that drug selection and dosage set forth in this text are in accordance with the current recommendations and practice at the time of publication. However, in view of ongoing research, changes in government regulations, and the constant flow of information relating to drug therapy and drug reactions, the reader is urged to check the package insert for each drug for any change in indications and dosage and for added warnings and precautions. This is particularly important when the recommended agent is a new or infrequently employed drug.

Some drugs and medical devices presented in this publication have Food and Drug Administration (FDA) clearance for limited use in restricted research settings. It is the responsibility of the health care provider to ascertain the FDA status of each drug or device planned for use in their clinical practice.

To purchase additional copies of this book, call our customer service department at **(800) 638-3030** or fax orders to **(301) 223-2320**. International customers should call **(301) 223-2300**.

Visit Lippincott Williams & Wilkins on the Internet: **http://www.lww.com**. Lippincott Williams & Wilkins customer service representatives are available from 8:30 am to 6:00 pm, EST.

Preface

Introduction to the Course

Welcome to the National Academy of Sports Medicine's (NASM's) Essentials of Sports Performance Training home-study course. At NASM, our mission is to help athletes accomplish all of their sports performance goals. We aim to give Sports Performance Professionals an integrated approach to sports performance, allowing them to guide others toward decreasing their risk of injury and maximizing performance. Our educational continuum employs an easy-to-use, systematic approach to apply scientific, clinically accepted concepts.

How to Use This Study Guide?

This study guide is designed to help you master the basic concepts presented in the course. This study guide provides students with a way to evaluate their knowledge, strengths, and weaknesses through an interactive review process.

Simply follow the student planner in this study guide. For each week, read the corresponding sections and complete the assignments listed. By following the student planner, you will stay focused on key areas and make studying simple. The student planner has been carefully organized to break down scientific concepts into manageable sections. You may move at a faster pace if you desire, but we suggest following the student planner to ensure proper mastery of all concepts.

Study Tips

The most important characteristic for students to possess is a deep and passionate desire to learn. That said, the following tips should help maximize the time spent on the course materials.

1. *Pace yourself.* You will be spending time watching Flash presentations and video demonstrations as well as reading the course text. Allow yourself enough time to get through the materials and thoroughly comprehend the information before progressing within the course.

2. *Schedule your study time.* Use the student planner provided in this study guide, and fill in your specific study dates. Make sure to stick to them. This will ensure a reasonable timeframe for completing your work and examination.

3. *Read and re-read.* When reviewing the course text, scan the information once to obtain an overview of the material. Then, go back and read the information thoroughly.

4. *Think about it.* Stop frequently as you review course material to consider the concepts presented. Ask yourself how and when you can apply the techniques and information covered.

5. *Lighten up.* Use a highlighter to accent important concepts and information or areas that may require additional review and practice.

6. *Do the exercises.* For the chapters that include exercises, NASM strongly recommends going through the exercises provided in those sections after you have completed your reading.

7. *Practice, practice, practice.* Remember that regular review and application of these principles are essential to your success. Apply what you have learned at every opportunity to help improve your techniques.

Getting Help

At NASM, your success is our success. We want to help in every way we can. The NASM staff is available to offer any assistance you may need throughout the course of your program. Whether you have technical or educational questions, we are available by phone and e-mail 8:00 a.m. to 5:00 p.m. (PST), Monday through Friday. Please call our toll-free number at 800.460.NASM or e-mail us questions at www.nasm.org.

Success Plan

You have 120 days from your registration (date of purchase) to fully complete the course and take the final examination. Be sure to schedule your time accordingly! Use the student planner to stay focused and track your progress. The student planner follows a 16-week reading and study plan. It is recommended that you do not take much time off between study sessions so that you will retain the material.

Average amounts of study time each day fall between one half to a full hour. Make sure that you have about 45 minutes to study on any given day. Sticking to the student planner will also give you ample time to prepare for the final examination before the 120-day expiration.

STUDENT PLANNER

Study Week	Completion Date	Course Materials	Assignment
Week 1	_____ *Fill in today's date*	Chapter 1	• Become familiar with all study materials and online format • Read Chapter 1 • Watch Chapter 1 presentation • Complete Chapter 1 exercises in the study guide
Week 2	_____ *Date*	Chapter 2	• Read Chapter 2 • Watch Chapter 2 presentation • Complete Chapter 2 exercises in the study guide
Week 3	_____ *Date*	Chapter 3	• Read Chapter 3 • Watch Chapter 3 presentation • Complete Chapter 3 exercises in the study guide • Practical application: practice sports performance assessments
Week 4	_____ *Date*	Chapter 4	• Read Chapter 4 • Watch Chapter 4 presentation • Complete Chapter 4 exercises in the study guide • Practical application: practice flexibility exercises
Week 5	_____ *Date*	Chapter 5	• Read Chapter 5 • Watch Chapter 5 presentation • Complete Chapter 5 exercises in the study guide • Practical application: practice cardiorespiratory programs
Week 6	_____ *Date*	Chapter 6	• Read Chapter 6 • Watch Chapter 6 presentation • Complete Chapter 6 exercises in the study guide • Practical application: practice core exercises
Week 7	_____ *Date*	Chapter 7	• Read Chapter 7 • Watch Chapter 7 presentation • Complete Chapter 7 exercises in the study guide • Practical application: practice balance exercises
Week 8	_____ *Date*	Chapter 8	• Read Chapter 8 • Watch Chapter 8 presentation • Complete Chapter 8 exercises in the study guide • Practical application: practice plyometric exercises
Week 9	_____ *Date*	Chapter 9	• Read Chapter 9 • Watch Chapter 9 presentation • Complete Chapter 9 exercises in the study guide • Practical application: practice SAQ exercises
Week 10	_____ *Date*	Chapter 10	• Read Chapter 10 • Watch Chapter 10 presentation • Complete Chapter 10 exercises in the study guide • Practical application: practice resistance exercises
Week 11	_____ *Date*	Chapter 11	• Read Chapter 11 • Watch Chapter 11 presentation • Complete Chapter 11 exercises in the study guide • Practical application: practice Olympic lifting exercises

STUDENT PLANNER (*Continued*)

Study Week	Completion Date	Course Materials	Assignment
Week 12	_____ *Date*	Chapter 12	• Read Chapter 12 • Watch Chapter 12 presentation • Complete Chapter 12 exercises in the study guide
Week 13	_____ *Date*	Chapter 13	• Read Chapter 13 • Watch Chapter 13 presentation • Complete Chapter 13 exercises in the study guide
Week 14	_____ *Date*	Chapter 14 Chapter 15	• Read Chapter 14 • Watch Chapter 14 presentation • Complete Chapter 14 exercises in the study guide • Read Chapter 15 • Watch Chapter 15 presentation • Complete Chapter 15 exercises in the study guide
Week 15	_____ *Date*	Chapter 16	• Read Chapter 16 • Watch Chapter 16 presentation • Complete Chapter 16 exercises in the study guide
Week 16	_____ *Date*	Review Final Examination	• Review your notes and highlights in text • Review all chapter exercises • Take the online practice examination (www.nasm.org) • After you have finished, review any sections that you had trouble with • Take the final examination and become an NASM Performance Enhancement Specialist

Contents

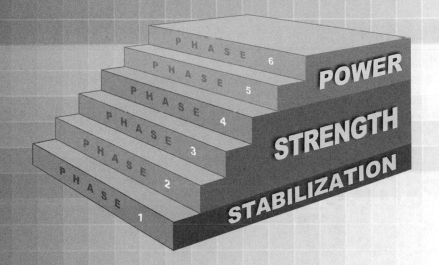

SECTION I

Principles and Concepts of Human Movement Science

CHAPTER 1

The Essentials of Integrated Training

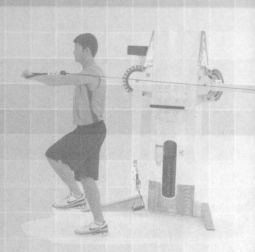

▌ EXERCISE 1-1   Essential Vocabulary

PURPOSE: To gain an understanding of key terms utilized in Chapter 1 of the textbook.

INSTRUCTIONS: Match the terms with their proper definitions.

VOCABULARY WORDS

1. _____ Stretch-shortening cycle

2. _____ Altered reciprocal inhibition

3. _____ Synergistic dominance

4. _____ Flexibility

5. _____ Core

6. _____ Neuromuscular efficiency

7. _____ Strength

DEFINITIONS

A. The ability of the neuromuscular system to exert force against resistance.

B. When synergists compensate for a weak or inhibited prime mover in an attempt to maintain force production and functional movement patterns.

C. When a tight muscle causes decreased neural drive to its functional antagonist.

D. The ability of the Human Movement System to allow agonists, antagonists, synergists, and stabilizers to work synergistically to produce force, reduce force, and dynamically stabilize the entire Human Movement System.

E. Provides intersegmental stability, deceleration, and force production during athletic activities.

F. Ability of the Human Movement System to have optimum range of motion as well as neuromuscular control throughout that range of motion.

G. An active stretch (eccentric contraction) of a muscle followed by an immediate shortening (concentric contraction) of that same muscle.

EXERCISE 1-2	**Short Answer**

INSTRUCTIONS: Answer the following question in one or two sentences.

1. What is the definition of integrated training?

_____

_____

_____

EXERCISE 1-3	**True/False**

1. Traditional strength and conditioning programs primarily focus on absolute or maximum strength gains in isolated muscles (chiefly the prime movers) throughout single planes of motion.

   TRUE   FALSE

2. Muscles can have some anatomical individuality, but they lack functional individuality.

   TRUE   FALSE

3. The central nervous system is designed to optimize the selection of muscle synergies to perform integrated movement patterns in all three planes of motion.

   TRUE   FALSE

4. Training only in the sagittal plane will not effectively prepare your athlete's muscles to be strong in all three planes of motion.

   TRUE   FALSE

5. Allowing an athlete to perform exercises with poor posture may result in the development of muscle imbalances and possible injury.

   TRUE   FALSE

6. Muscle overactivity, adaptive muscle shortening, or both can cause altered reciprocal inhibition and synergistic dominance.

   TRUE   FALSE

7. An integrated sports performance training program primarily focuses on uniplanar training and concentric force production.

   TRUE   FALSE

8. Components of an integrated sports performance training program include flexibility, core, balance, plyometrics, speed, agility, quickness, resistance training, and sports-specific cardiorespiratory conditioning.

   TRUE   FALSE

9. There are many types of strength including maximal strength, relative strength, strength endurance, speed strength, stabilization strength, and functional strength.

   TRUE   FALSE

10. The following are proper exercise progressions: fast to slow, complex to simple, unknown to known, high force to low force, eyes closed to eyes open, dynamic to static.

    TRUE   FALSE

CHAPTER 2

Introduction to Human Movement Science

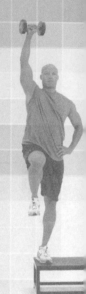

EXERCISE 2-1   **Essential Vocabulary**

PURPOSE: To gain an understanding of key terms utilized in Chapter 2 of the textbook.

INSTRUCTIONS: Match the terms with their proper definitions.

VOCABULARY WORDS

1. _____ Biomechanics

2. _____ Force

3. _____ Rotary motion

4. _____ Torque

5. _____ Agonist

6. _____ Antagonists

7. _____ Synergists

8. _____ Stabilizers

9. _____ Motor behavior

10. _____ Motor control

11. _____ Motor learning

12. _____ Motor development

13. _____ Internal feedback

14. _____ External feedback

DEFINITIONS

A. Movement of bones around joints.

B. Muscles that assist prime movers during functional movement patterns.

C. Muscles that act as prime movers.

D. A force that produces rotation.

E. Applies the principles of physics to quantitatively study how forces interact within a living body.

F. Feedback provided by some external source.

G. An influence applied by one object to another, which results in an acceleration or a deceleration of the second object.

H. Muscles that act in direct opposition to prime movers.

I. Feedback used after the completion of a movement to help inform the client about the outcome of his or her performance.

J. The change in motor behavior over time throughout the lifespan.

15. _____ Knowledge of results

16. _____ Knowledge of performance

K. Integration of motor control processes through practice and experience leading to a relatively permanent change in the capacity to produce skilled movements.

L. Human Movement System response to internal and external environmental stimuli.

M. Muscles that support or stabilize the body while the prime movers and the synergists perform the movement patterns.

N. Sensory information provided by the body via length-tension relationships, force-couple relationships, and arthrokinematics to monitor movement and the environment.

O. The study of posture and movements with the involved structures and mechanisms used by the central nervous system to assimilate and integrate sensory information with previous experiences.

P. Feedback that provides information about the quality of the movement during exercise.

EXERCISE 2-2   Knowledge of Terms

INSTRUCTIONS: Use the following terms to fill in the blanks below.

Transverse plane

Sagittal plane

Concentric contraction

Frontal plane

Pronation

Supination

Isometric contraction

Eccentric contraction

1. The _____ _____ bisects the body into right and left halves and primarily includes flexion and extension movements.

2. The _____ _____ bisects the body into front and back halves and primarily includes abduction and adduction of the limbs (relative to the trunk), lateral flexion in the spine, and eversion and inversion of the foot and ankle complex.

3. The _____ _____ bisects the body to create upper and lower halves and primarily includes internal rotation and external rotation for the limbs, right and left rotation for the head and trunk, and radioulnar pronation and supination.

4. _____ is a multiplanar, synchronized joint motion that occurs with eccentric muscle function.

5. _____ is a multiplanar, synchronized joint motion that occurs with concentric muscle function.

6. An _____ _____ occurs when a muscle develops tension while lengthening; the muscle lengthens because the contractile force is less than the resistive force.

7. An _____ _____ occurs when the contractile force is equal to the resistive force leading to no visible change in the muscle length.

8. A _____ _____ occurs when the contractile force is greater than the resistive force, resulting in shortening of the muscle and visible joint movement.

EXERCISE 2-3   Multiple Choice

1. The lateral subsystem consists of which muscle groups?
   a. Gluteus medius, tensor fascia latae, adductor complex, quadratus lumborum
   b. Anterior tibialis, posterior tibialis, erector spinae, posterior deltoid
   c. Pectoralis major, rhomboids, trapezius, adductor complex
   d. Rectus abdominus, external oblique, internal oblique

2. What are the major muscle groups of the deep longitudinal subsystem?
   a. Pectoralis major, pectoralis minor, triceps brachii
   b. Erector spinae, thoracolumbar fascia, sacrotuberous ligament, biceps femoris, and peroneus longus
   c. Upper, middle, and lower trapezius
   d. Gastrocnemius, soleus, peroneus longus, peroneus brevis

3. What are the prime contributors to the anterior oblique subsystem?
   a. Gluteus maximus, gluteus medius, gluteus minimus
   b. Quadriceps, hamstrings, gluteus maximus
   c. Internal and external oblique muscles, the adductor complex, and hip external rotators
   d. Multifidus, diaphragm, erector spinae, psoas

4. Which subsystem works synergistically with the deep longitudinal subsystem and consists of the gluteus maximus, thoracolumbar fascia, and contralateral latissimus dorsi.
   a. Deep longitudinal subsystem
   b. Anterior oblique subsystem
   c. Lateral subsystem
   d. Posterior oblique subsystem

5. The joint support system of the lumbo-pelvic-hip complex includes the
   a. transverse abdominis, multifidus, internal oblique, diaphragm, pelvic floor muscles.
   b. rectus abdominis, external oblique, latissimus dorsi.
   c. rectus femoris, bicep femoris, psoas.
   d. pectoralis minor, erector spinae, levator scapulae, sternocleidomastoid.

6. What is the cumulative neural input from sensory afferents to the central nervous system?
   a. Sensation
   b. Perception
   c. Proprioception
   d. Force-couple relationships

7. What part of the nervous system is designed to optimize muscle synergies?
   a. Peripheral
   b. Autonomic
   c. Parasympathetic
   d. Central

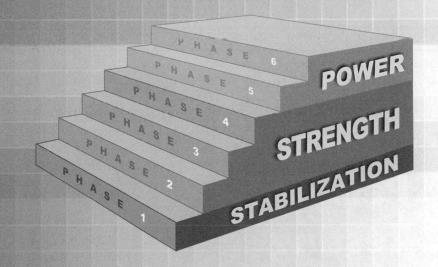

SECTION 2

Human Performance Testing and Evaluation

CHAPTER 3

Sports Performance Testing

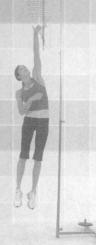

EXERCISE 3-1   **Essential Vocabulary**

PURPOSE: To gain an understanding of key terms used in Chapter 3 of the textbook.

INSTRUCTIONS: Match the terms with their proper definitions.

VOCABULARY WORDS

1. _____ Objective information

2. _____ Structural efficiency

3. _____ Functional efficiency

4. _____ Functional strength

DEFINITIONS

A. The alignment of the musculoskeletal system, which allows our center of gravity to be maintained over a base of support.

B. The ability of the neuromuscular system to monitor and manipulate movement during functional tasks using the least amount of energy, creating the least amount of stress on the kinetic chain.

C. The ability of the neuromuscular system to contract eccentrically, isometrically, and concentrically in all three planes of motion.

D. Measurable data about a client's physical state such as body composition, movement, and cardiovascular ability.

EXERCISE 3-2   True/False

1. Designing an individualized, sports performance program can be properly accomplished only by having an understanding of an athlete's goals, needs, and abilities.

   TRUE   FALSE

2. The first step in the sports performance assessment is to gather the athlete's personal medical history.

   TRUE   FALSE

3. The PAR-Q is directed toward detecting any possible cardiorespiratory dysfunction, such as coronary heart disease, and is a good starting point for gathering personal background information concerning a prospective athlete's cardiorespiratory function.

   TRUE   FALSE

4. Ankle sprains have been shown to decrease the neural control to the gluteus medius and gluteus maximus muscles.

   TRUE   FALSE

5. Noncontact knee injuries are often the result of ankle and/or hip dysfunctions.

   TRUE   FALSE

6. Low-back injuries can cause an increase in neural control to stabilizing muscles of the core, resulting in additional stabilization of the spine.

   TRUE   FALSE

7. Shoulder injuries may cause altered neural control of the rotator cuff muscles, leading to instability of the shoulder joint during functional activities.

   TRUE   FALSE

8. It is the role of a Sports Performance Professional to administer, prescribe, or educate on the usage and effects of physician-prescribed medications.

   TRUE   FALSE

9. Basic categories of objective information include physiological assessments, postural assessments, and performance assessments.

   TRUE   FALSE

10. β-Blockers typically increase an athlete's heart rate and blood pressure.

    TRUE   FALSE

EXERCISE 3-3   Multiple Choice

1. Blood pressure measurements consist of systolic and diastolic readings. Normal diastolic pressure ranges from

   a. 80 to 85 mm Hg.
   b. 90 to 95 mm Hg.
   c. 96 to 100 mm Hg.
   d. 120 to 130 mm Hg.

2. All of the following are examples of a physiological assessment EXCEPT
   a. blood pressure.
   b. medical questionnaire.
   c. resting heart rate.
   d. circumference measurement.

3. All of the following help determine an athlete's body-fat percentage EXCEPT
   a. skin-fold measurement.
   b. underwater weighing.
   c. bioelectrical impedance.
   d. body mass index.

4. The Durnin formula's four sites of skin-fold measurement are as follows:
   a. Biceps, triceps, subscapular, iliac crest
   b. Calf, thigh, abdomen, subscapular
   c. Biceps, triceps, abdomen, calf
   d. Calf, thigh, chest, abdomen

5. Ideal functional posture maintains the structural integrity and optimum alignment of each component of the Human Movement System, promoting all of the following EXCEPT
   a. optimum length-tension relationships.
   b. optimum force-couple relationships.
   c. optimum synergistic dominance.
   d. optimum joint arthrokinematics.

6. Transitional postural assessments include all of the following EXCEPT
   a. overhead squat assessment.
   b. single-leg squat assessment.
   c. landing error scoring system.
   d. pulling assessment.

7. Knee valgus during the overhead squat test is influenced by all of the following EXCEPT
   a. decreased hip abductor and hip external rotation strength.
   b. increased hip adductor activity.
   c. restricted ankle dorsiflexion.
   d. restricted ankle eversion.

8. All of the following muscles are implicated as possibly overactive when an athlete's low-back arches during the overhead squat assessment EXCEPT
   a. gluteus maximus.
   b. hip flexor complex.
   c. erector spinae.
   d. latissimus dorsi.

9. All of the following muscles are implicated as possibly underactive when an athlete's knee moves inward during the single-leg squat assessment EXCEPT
   a. gluteus medius.
   b. adductor complex.
   c. vastus medialis oblique.
   d. gluteus maximus.

10. All of the following muscles are implicated as possibly overactive when an athlete's head migrates forward during the pushing assessment EXCEPT
    a. upper trapezius.
    b. sternocleidomastoid.
    c. deep cervical flexors.
    d. levator scapulae.

11. All of the following are stability assessments EXCEPT

    a. Double-Leg Lowering Test.
    b. Single-leg STAR Balance Excursion Test.
    c. 185-lb Bench Press.
    d. Sorensen Erector Spinae Test.

12. Which of the following assessments measures muscular endurance of the pulling muscles of the upper body?

    a. Upper-Extremity Strength Assessment: Bench Press
    b. 185-lb Bench Press: Basketball
    c. Push-Ups
    d. Pull-Ups

EXERCISE 3-4   Matching

INSTRUCTIONS: Answer the following questions, referring to the images below.

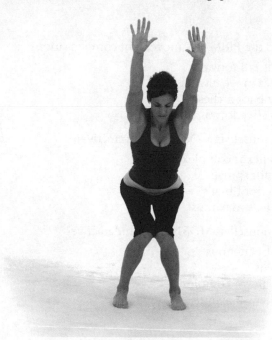

1. What is the PRIMARY movement compensation?

    a. Arms fall forward
    b. Knees move inward
    c. Low-back arches
    d. Excessive forward lean

2. Which muscle is MOST likely overactive?

    a. Medial hamstring
    b. Medial gastrocnemius
    c. Adductor complex
    d. Gluteus medius

3. Which muscle is MOST likely underactive?

    a. Gluteus medius
    b. Tensor fascia latae
    c. Adductor complex
    d. Biceps femoris (short head)

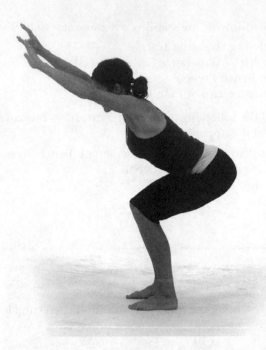

4. What is the PRIMARY movement compensation?

   a. Arms fall forward
   b. Knees move inward
   c. Low-back arches
   d. Excessive forward lean

5. Which muscle is MOST likely overactive?

   a. Hip flexor complex
   b. Erector spinae
   c. Anterior tibialis
   d. Gluteus maximus

6. Which muscle is MOST likely underactive?

   a. Gastrocnemius
   b. Soleus
   c. Hip flexor complex
   d. Gluteus maximus

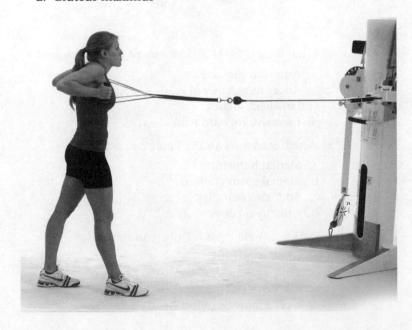

7. What is the PRIMARY movement compensation?

    a. Shoulders elevate
    b. Knees move inward
    c. Low-back rounds
    d. Excessive forward lean

8. Which muscle is MOST likely overactive?

    a. Rotator cuff
    b. Upper trapezius
    c. Lower trapezius
    d. Rhomboids

9. Which muscle is MOST likely underactive?

    a. Lower trapezius
    b. Upper trapezius
    c. Sternocleidomastoid
    d. Levator scapulae

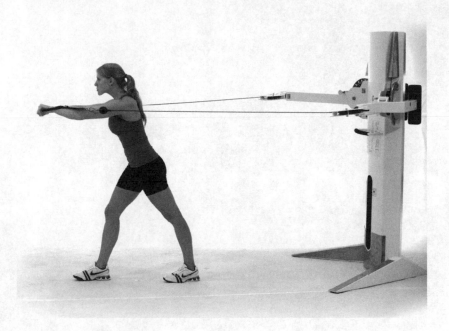

10. What is the PRIMARY movement compensation?

    a. Shoulders elevate
    b. Knees move inward
    c. Low-back rounds
    d. Forward head

11. Which muscle is MOST likely overactive?

    a. Rotator cuff
    b. Deep cervical flexors
    c. Gluteus maximus
    d. Sternocleidomastoid

12. Which muscle is MOST likely underactive?

    a. Deep cervical flexors
    b. Levator scapulae
    c. Sternocleidomastoid
    d. Scalenes

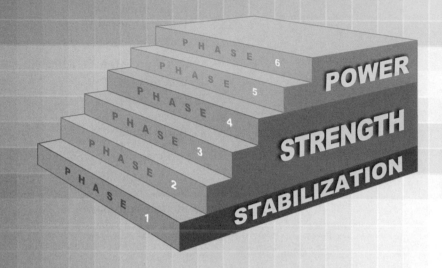

SECTION 3

Components of Integrated Performance Training

CHAPTER 4

Flexibility Training for Performance Enhancement

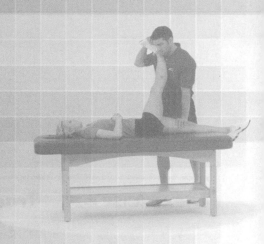

EXERCISE 4-1   Essential Vocabulary

PURPOSE: To gain an understanding of key terms used in Chapter 4 of the textbook.

INSTRUCTIONS: Match the terms with their proper definitions.

VOCABULARY WORDS

1. _____ Arthrokinetic dysfunction

2. _____ Endomysium

3. _____ Perimysium

4. _____ Epimysium

5. _____ Cumulative injury cycle

6. _____ Muscle spindles

7. _____ Golgi tendon organs

8. _____ Joint mechanoreceptors

9. _____ Atrophy

10. _____ Rate coding

11. _____ Sarcopenia

12. _____ Elasticity

DEFINITIONS

A. The outermost layer of muscle (fascia) binding entire fascicles together.

B. A process whereby an injury will induce inflammation, muscle spasm, adhesions, altered neuromuscular control, and muscle imbalances.

C. The biomechanical dysfunction in two articular partners that lead to abnormal joint movement (arthrokinematics) and proprioception.

D. Major sensory organs of the muscle sensitive to change in length and rate of length change.

E. Located within the musculotendinous junction, and are sensitive to tension, and rate of tension change.

F. The sheath that binds groups of muscle fibers into fasciculi.

G. Located in joints throughout the fibrous capsule and ligaments and signal joint position, movement, and pressure changes.

13. _____ Davis's Law

14. _____ Wolff's Law

H. The innermost fascial layer that encases individual muscle fibers.

I. A decrease in muscle fiber numbers.

J. The loss in muscle fiber size.

K. The spring-like behavior of connective tissue that enables the tissue to return to its original shape or size when forces are removed.

L. Soft tissue models along the lines of stress.

M. Bone in a healthy person or animal will adapt to the loads it is placed under.

N. The rate at which any individual nerve fiber transmits impulses per unit of time.

EXERCISE 4-2   True/False

1. Regardless of the goal, always begin a flexibility program with movement assessments such as the overhead squat and/or the single-leg squat to help determine the muscles that need to be focused on in a flexibility program.

   TRUE   FALSE

2. When used in a warm-up, static stretching should be used only on areas that the assessments have determined are weak/underactive.

   TRUE   FALSE

3. During the cool-down, static stretching should be used to return muscles to normal resting lengths focusing on the major muscles utilized during the workout.

   TRUE   FALSE

4. Proprioceptive neuromuscular facilitation/neuromuscular stretching techniques have been shown to provide an acute increase in range of motion and assist in teaching proper reciprocal inhibition and neuromuscular efficiency.

   TRUE   FALSE

5. Static stretching, if incorporated before a strength workout or as a warm-up prior to competition, should be followed by active-isolated and/or dynamic stretching to improve neuromuscular efficiency.

   TRUE   FALSE

6. Static stretching is contraindicated prior to all activities requiring maximal efforts even if muscle imbalances are present.

   TRUE   FALSE

7. Active-isolated and/or dynamic stretching can be used as a warm-up by themselves if no muscle imbalances are present.

   TRUE   FALSE

8. A proper flexibility program would also require implementation of a corrective strengthening program to enhance range of motion.

   TRUE   FALSE

9. When one segment in the Human Movement System is out of alignment and is not functioning optimally, predictable patterns of dysfunction develop and initiate the cumulative injury cycle.

   TRUE   FALSE

10. Optimal neuromuscular efficiency of the Human Movement System can exist only if all components (muscular, articular, and neural) function optimally and interdependently.
    TRUE   FALSE

EXERCISE 4-3   Short Answer

INSTRUCTIONS: Answer the following question in a few sentences.

1. What are the causes of muscle imbalances?

    _____

    _____

    _____

EXERCISE 4-4   Multiple Choice

1. Flexibility is the normal _____ of all soft tissues that allow full range of motion at a joint.
    a. viscosity
    b. extensibility
    c. plasticity
    d. contractility

2. Static stretching is a form of
    a. corrective flexibility.
    b. active flexibility.
    c. dynamic flexibility.
    d. passive flexibility.

3. Connective tissue is primarily composed of elastic and _____ fibers.
    a. plastin
    b. myosin
    c. collagenous
    d. actin

4. The residual or permanent change in connective tissue length due to tissue elongation best describes
    a. plasticity.
    b. viscoelasticity.
    c. viscosity.
    d. eccentricity.

5. Slow deformation and imperfect recovery of connective tissue best describe
    a. plasticity.
    b. viscoelasticity.
    c. viscosity.
    d. eccentricity.

6. Connective tissue surrounding neural tissue is self-innervated by the
    a. sciatic nerve.
    b. neurovascular triad.

    c. mesonerium.

    d. nervi nervorum.

7. Each sarcomere is made up of _____, which includes overlapping thick (myosin) and thin (actin) contractile proteins.

    a. sarcomere

    b. fascicle

    c. myofilaments

    d. endomysium

8. Self-innervation and an abundant blood supply allow the connective tissue of the nerve to be very:

    a. Pain sensitive

    b. Pain resistant

    c. Tight

    d. Nerves do not receive blood

9. An integrated training and flexibility program can delay physical changes associated with aging such as muscle atrophy and

    a. soft tissue hydration.

    b. soft tissue dehydration.

    c. neural hypertrophy.

    d. muscle hypertrophy.

10. Static stretching and self-myofascial release forms of stretching use the principle of _____ to improve soft tissue extensibility.

    a. autogenic inhibition

    b. reciprocal inhibition

    c. muscle hypertrophy

    d. excitation-contraction coupling

CHAPTER 5

Cardiorespiratory Training for Performance Enhancement

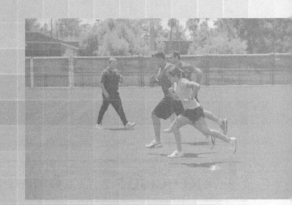

EXERCISE 5-1   Essential Vocabulary

PURPOSE: The purpose of this exercise is to have an understanding of key terms utilized in Chapter 5.

INSTRUCTIONS: Match the terms with their proper definitions.

VOCABULARY WORDS

1. _____ Glycogen
2. _____ Interval training
3. _____ Pulmonary ventilation
4. _____ Excess postexercise oxygen consumption
5. _____ Systolic pressure
6. _____ Diastolic pressure
7. _____ Cardiac output
8. _____ Respiratory quotient
9. _____ Anaerobic threshold
10. _____ Stroke volume

DEFINITIONS

A. The process that brings oxygen from the air, across the alveolar membrane, and into the blood to be carried by hemoglobin.

B. The heart pumping blood out of the left ventricle into the aorta, distending it and creating pressure on the vascular wall.

C. The amount of pressure in the arterial system needed to keep blood vessels open during the relaxation phase of the cardiac cycle.

D. The amount of blood the heart pumps per minute.

E. A large molecule stored in the liver and made up of chains of glucose.

F. The amount of carbon dioxide (CO_2) expired divided by the amount of oxygen (O_2) consumed and measured during rest or at steady state of exercise using a metabolic analyzer.

G. Training at different intensities for certain periods of time in a given workout.

H. The metabolic rate of an individual following exercise or activity.

I. When the body can no longer produce enough energy for working muscles solely through aerobic metabolism, leading to an increase of energy production through anaerobic metabolism.

J. The amount of blood pumped with each contraction of the ventricles.

EXERCISE 5-2   True/False

1. Of the various components that comprise an athlete's total physical fitness program, cardiorespiratory endurance is probably the most misunderstood and underrated.

   TRUE   FALSE

2. Without a proper cardiorespiratory base, an athlete's performance may decrease over time opening the door for underperformance and possible injury.

   TRUE   FALSE

3. The heart rate of a well-trained aerobic athlete can beat as few as 40 times a minute.

   TRUE   FALSE

4. The movement of oxygen and carbon dioxide into and out of the circulatory system takes place through diffusion.

   TRUE   FALSE

5. Resting cardiac output is typically around 6 L/min at rest and about 20–25 L/min during maximum exercise, but for the aerobic elite may be more than 40 L/min.

   TRUE   FALSE

6. The oxidative system involves only the respiratory and cardiovascular systems.

   TRUE   FALSE

7. Anaerobic energy pathways are the main source of energy for low-intensity, long-duration activities.

   TRUE   FALSE

8. One method to minimize lactic acid production while enhancing lactic acid removal during exercise is through a combination of high-intensity interval training and prolonged submaximal training.

   TRUE   FALSE

9. At the onset of exercise, the oxidative system is the first active bioenergetic pathway that gives way to ATP-CP and then to glycolysis energy production.

   TRUE   FALSE

10. Sprinting primarily utilizes the oxidative system.

    TRUE   FALSE

EXERCISE 5-3   Short Answer

INSTRUCTIONS: Answer the following questions in a few sentences.

1. Briefly describe a Phase 1 Base Training program.

_____

_____

_____

2. Briefly describe a Phase 2 Interval Training program.

_____

_____

_____

3. Briefly describe the function of Phases 3 through 5 of a cardiorespiratory conditioning program.

_____

_____

_____

4. What are some obvious signs and symptoms of overtraining?

_____

_____

_____

CHAPTER 6

Core Training Concepts for Performance Enhancement

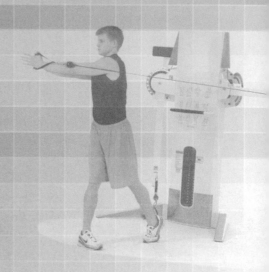

EXERCISE 6-1   ## Essential Vocabulary

PURPOSE: To gain an understanding of key terms utilized in Chapter 6.

INSTRUCTIONS: Match the terms with their proper definitions.

VOCABULARY WORDS

1. _____ Movement system

2. _____ Core power exercises

3. _____ Core stability

4. _____ Local core stabilizers

5. _____ Global stabilizers

6. _____ Core stabilization exercises

7. _____ Core strength exercises

8. _____ Bracing

DEFINITIONS

A. Often referred as neuromuscular efficiency of the core. But more accurately described as lumbo-pelvic-hip complex (LPHC) stability composed of local or intersegmental stability (local stabilization system), global stability (global stabilization system), and global mobility.

B. Muscles that attach directly to the vertebrae and are responsible for intervertebral/ intersegmental stability and work to limit excessive compressive, shear, and rotational forces between spinal segments.

C. Muscles that attach from the pelvis to the spine and act to transfer loads between the upper extremity and lower extremity and provide stability between the pelvis and spine.

D. Muscles that attach the spine and/or pelvis to the extremities and are primarily responsible for concentric force production and eccentric deceleration during dynamic activities.

9. _____ Drawing-in maneuver

10. _____ Core

E. Exercises that involve little to no motion through the spine and pelvis. These exercises are designed to improve neuromuscular efficiency and intervertebral stability by focusing on the local stabilization system.

F. Exercises that involve dynamic eccentric and concentric movements of the spine through a full range of motion while performing neuromechanical activation techniques (drawing-in and bracing).

G. Exercises designed to improve the rate of force production of the core musculature preparing an athlete to stabilize and to generate force dynamically at more functionally applicable speeds.

H. A maneuver used to recruit the local core stabilizers by pulling the navel in toward the spine.

I. Contraction of the abdominals, lower back, and buttock muscles at the same time.

J. The structures that make up the LPHC.

EXERCISE 6-2   Matching

INSTRUCTIONS: Answer the following questions, referring to the images below.

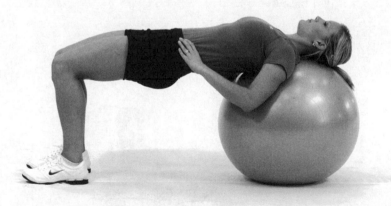

1. What type of core exercise is illustrated above?
   a. Core stabilization
   b. Core strength
   c. Core power

2. Which phase(s) of the OPT™ model would this exercise be most appropriate for?
   a. Phase 1
   b. Phases 2 and 3
   c. Phase 4
   d. Phases 5 and 6

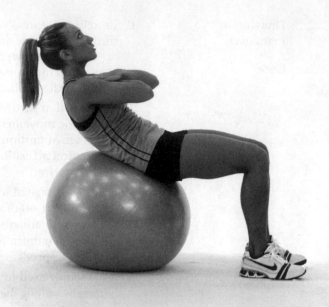

3. What type of core exercise is illustrated above?

   a. Core stabilization

   b. Core strength

   c. Core power

4. Which phase(s) of the OPT model would this exercise be most appropriate for?

   a. Phase 1

   b. Phases 2, 3, and 4

   c. Phase 5

   d. Phase 6

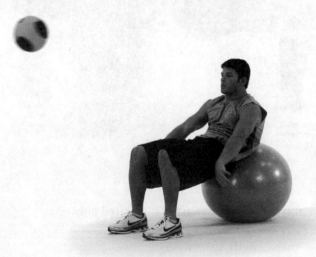

5. What type of core exercise is illustrated above?

   a. Core stabilization

   b. Core strength

   c. Core power

6. Which phase(s) of the OPT model would this exercise be most appropriate for?
   a. Phase 1
   b. Phase 2
   c. Phases 3 and 4
   d. Phases 5 and 6

EXERCISE 6-3   # True/False

1. The core operates as an integrated functional unit enabling the entire LPHC to work synergistically to produce force concentrically, decelerate force eccentrically, and stabilize against abnormal compressive, torsional, and shear forces isometrically.
   TRUE   FALSE

2. If the extremity muscles are strong and the core is weak, there will be insufficient forces moving throughout the Human Movement System for efficient movements.
   TRUE   FALSE

3. A weak core is a fundamental problem inherent to inefficient movement that may lead to predictable patterns of injury.
   TRUE   FALSE

4. The primary muscles that make up the movement system include the transverse abdominus, internal oblique, multifidus, pelvic floor musculature, and diaphragm.
   TRUE   FALSE

5. The thoracolumbar fascia is noncontractile but can be engaged dynamically because of the contractile tissues that attach to it.
   TRUE   FALSE

6. The muscles that attach to the thoracolumbar fascia include the rectus femoris, biceps femoris, vastus lateralis, and vastus medialis oblique.
   TRUE   FALSE

7. The increase in intra-abdominal pressure results in elevation of the diaphragm and contraction of pelvic floor musculature while also assisting in providing inter-segmental stabilization to the core.
   TRUE   FALSE

8. Several authors have found increased firing, hypertrophy, and force production of the transverse abdominus, internal oblique, and multifidus in individuals with chronic low-back pain.
   TRUE   FALSE

9. It has also been demonstrated that individuals with low-back pain have altered spinal proprioception.
   TRUE   FALSE

10. Performing spinal stabilization exercises may improve vertical jump and agility measures and enhance vertical takeoff velocity.
    TRUE   FALSE

CHAPTER 7

Balance Training Concepts for Performance Enhancement

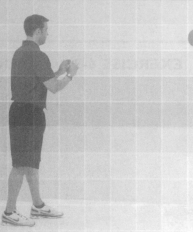

EXERCISE 7-1   **Essential Vocabulary**

PURPOSE: To gain an understanding of key terms used in Chapter 7 of the textbook.

INSTRUCTIONS: Match the terms with their proper definitions.

VOCABULARY WORDS

1. _____ Kinesthesia
2. _____ Mechanoreceptors
3. _____ Balance
4. _____ Ruffini afferents
5. _____ Proprioception
6. _____ Golgi afferents
7. _____ Paciniform afferents
8. _____ Nociceptors
9. _____ Multisensory condition
10. _____ Controlled instability
11. _____ Dynamic joint stabilization

DEFINITIONS

A. The cumulative neural input to the central nervous system (CNS) from all mechanoreceptors that sense position and limb movement.

B. The ability to maintain the body's center of gravity within its base of support.

C. The conscious awareness of joint movement and joint position sense that results from proprioceptive input sent to the CNS.

D. Specialized neural receptors embedded in connective tissue that convert mechanical distortions of the tissue into neural codes to be conveyed to the CNS.

E. These receptors are mechanically sensitive to tissue stresses that are activated during extremes of extension and rotation.

F. These receptors are widely distributed around the joint capsule and surrounding periarticular tissue that are mechanically sensitive to local compression and tensile loading, especially at extreme ranges of motion.

G. High threshold, slowly adapting sensory receptors located in ligaments and menisci, mechanically sensitive to tensile loads and are most sensitive at the end ranges of motion.

H. Small-diameter afferents located primarily in articular tissue and are sensitive to mechanical deformation and pain.

I. The ability of the kinetic chain to stabilize a joint during movement.

J. A training environment that provides heightened stimulation to the proprioceptors and mechanoreceptors.

K. A training environment that is as unstable as can be SAFELY controlled for an individual.

▌EXERCISE 7-2   **True/False**

1. During times of instability, such as standing in an unstable environment, the activation of the stabilizing muscles precedes the force production of the prime movers.

   TRUE   FALSE

2. Injury to joints or corresponding muscles along the kinetic chain can result in a loss of appropriate feedback for maintaining balance.

   TRUE   FALSE

3. The apparently simple act of maintaining an athletic position during sport is actually a continuing process of minute adjustments to keep the athlete's center of gravity over his or her base of support.

   TRUE   FALSE

4. It is proposed that balance and postural control are accounted for by two main neurophysiological mechanisms: peripheral neural mechanisms and central processing.

   TRUE   FALSE

5. Maximal strength is more significant than visual, vestibular, and proprioceptive inputs for maintaining postural control and balance.

   TRUE   FALSE

6. The sensory afferent neurons that detect skin stretching also supply information about joint rotation.

   TRUE   FALSE

7. When stretching activates the muscle spindle, a sensory response is evoked and transmitted to the spinal cord, which in turn sends impulses back to the muscle producing relaxation of the agonist and synergistic muscle fibers.

   TRUE   FALSE

8. Sensory information regarding the length of the muscle and the rate of change in length is transmitted to the CNS by the Golgi tendon organ.

   TRUE   FALSE

9. The muscle spindle is primarily sensitive to tension development and rate of tension development in skeletal muscle.

TRUE   FALSE

10. Research postulates that the Golgi tendon organ functions as a protective mechanism to prevent overcontraction of the muscle.

TRUE   FALSE

EXERCISE 7-3   Short Answer

INSTRUCTIONS: Briefly answer the following question.

1. What is the scientific rationale for balance training and its importance in sports performance?

_____

_____

_____

EXERCISE 7-4   Matching

INSTRUCTIONS: Answer the following questions referring to the images below.

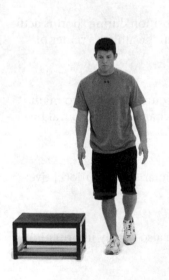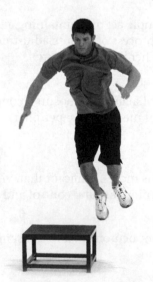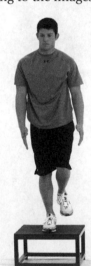

1. What type of balance exercise is illustrated above?

   a. Balance stabilization
   b. Balance strength
   c. Balance power

2. Which phase(s) of the OPT model would this exercise be most appropriate for?

   a. Phase 1
   b. Phases 2 and 3
   c. Phase 4
   d. Phases 5 and 6

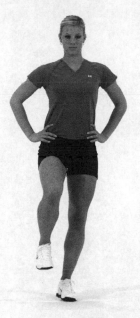

3. What type of balance exercise is illustrated above?

   a. Balance stabilization
   b. Balance strength
   c. Balance power

4. Which phase(s) of the OPT model would this exercise be most appropriate for?

   a. Phase 1
   b. Phases 2 and 3
   c. Phase 4
   d. Phases 5 and 6

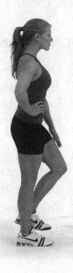
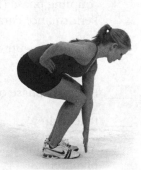

5. What type of balance exercise is illustrated above?

   a. Balance stabilization
   b. Balance strength
   c. Balance power

6. Which phase(s) of the OPT model would this exercise be most appropriate for?

   a. Phase 1
   b. Phases 2, 3, and 4
   c. Phase 5
   d. Phase 6

CHAPTER 8

Plyometric Training Concepts for Performance Enhancement

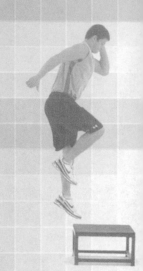

EXERCISE 8-1 **Essential Vocabulary**

PURPOSE: To gain an understanding of key terms used in Chapter 8 of the textbook.

INSTRUCTIONS: Match the terms with their proper definitions.

VOCABULARY WORDS

1. _____ Eccentric-concentric coupling phase (Integrated Performance Paradigm™)

2. _____ Rate of force production (power)

3. _____ Eccentric phase of plyometrics

4. _____ Rate coding

5. _____ Amortization phase of plyometrics

6. _____ Concentric phase of plyometrics

DEFINITIONS

A. The concept that states, in order to move with precision, forces must be loaded (eccentrically), stabilized (isometrically), and then unloaded/accelerated (concentrically).

B. The ability of muscles to exert maximal force output in a minimal amount of time.

C. This phase occurs immediately after the amortization phase of a plyometric exercise.

D. Motor unit firing frequency.

E. This phase increases muscle spindle activity by prestretching the muscle prior to activation.

F. This phase is the time between the end of the eccentric contraction and the initiation of the concentric contraction.

EXERCISE 8-2   True/False

1. Success in most functional activities depends on the speed at which muscular force is generated.
   TRUE   FALSE

2. The ultimate goal of plyometric training is to improve the reaction time of the muscle action spectrum.
   TRUE   FALSE

3. The speed of muscular exertion is limited by neuromuscular coordination.
   TRUE   FALSE

4. A slower eccentric phase takes optimum advantage of the myotatic stretch reflex resulting in greater force production.
   TRUE   FALSE

5. A prolonged amortization phase results in optimum neuromuscular efficiency and maximum utilization of elastic potential energy.
   TRUE   FALSE

6. When a load is applied to a joint, the elastic elements stretch and store potential energy prior to the contractile element contracting.
   TRUE   FALSE

7. When performing a vertical jump, the longer one waits at the end of the counter-movement before performing the jump, the higher the eventual jump height due to the ability to recover the stored elastic energy.
   TRUE   FALSE

EXERCISE 8-3   Multiple Choice

1. All of the following are true regarding plyometric training EXCEPT
   a. increase in motor unit recruitment.
   b. increase in resting heart rate.
   c. increase in motor learning.
   d. increase in rate of force production.

2. The three phases of plyometric training in order are _____, _____, _____.
   a. eccentric, amortization, concentric
   b. eccentric, concentric, amortization
   c. concentric, eccentric, amortization
   d. concentric, amortization, eccentric

3. The amortization phase is referred to as a(n) _____ delay.
   a. electrical
   b. mechanical
   c. electromechanical
   d. musculoskeletal

4. Decreasing sensitization of the Golgi tendon organ will help _____ force production.

   a. increase
   b. decrease
   c. sustain
   d. limit

5. Athletes with minimal experience using plyometrics should keep the ground contacts to less than ____ maximal efforts per session.

   a. 400
   b. 300
   c. 200
   d. 100

6. What type of exercise is the "squat jump with stabilization"?

   a. Plyometric stabilization
   b. Plyometric strength
   c. Plyometric power

7. Which phase(s) of the OPT model would be MOST appropriate for the "box jump-up with stabilization" exercise?

   a. Phase 1
   b. Phases 2, 3, and 4
   c. Phase 5
   d. Phase 6

8. What type of exercise is the "repeat squat jump"?

   a. Plyometric stabilization
   b. Plyometric strength
   c. Plyometric power

9. Which phase(s) of the OPT model would be MOST appropriate for the "repeat box jump-up" exercise?

   a. Phase 1
   b. Phases 2, 3, and 4
   c. Phase 5
   d. Phase 6

10. What type of exercise is the "depth-jump to sprinting"?

    a. Plyometric stabilization
    b. Plyometric strength
    c. Plyometric power

11. Which phase(s) of the OPT model would be MOST appropriate for the "hurdle jump to vertical jump" exercise?

    a. Phase 1
    b. Phases 2 and 3
    c. Phase 4
    d. Phases 5 and 6

CHAPTER 9

Speed Agility and Quickness Training for Performance Enhancement

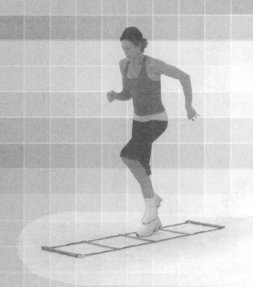

EXERCISE 9-1   Essential Vocabulary

PURPOSE: To gain an understanding of key terms used in Chapter 9 of the textbook.

INSTRUCTIONS: Match the terms with their proper definitions.

VOCABULARY WORDS

1. _____ Overspeed/assisted drills
2. _____ Joint mobility
3. _____ Force-velocity curve
4. _____ Stretch-shortening cycle
5. _____ Resisted speed drills
6. _____ Linear speed
7. _____ Stride rate
8. _____ Stride length
9. _____ Overstriding
10. _____ Front-side mechanics
11. _____ Back-side mechanics
12. _____ Agility

DEFINITIONS

A. When the force demands of an activity increase, the velocity output of the movement decreases.

B. A forced and rapid lengthening of a muscle immediately followed by a shortening of a muscle, creating an elastic "rubber-band-like" effect of energy release.

C. The ability of a joint to move through its natural, effective range of motion.

D. A type of training utilizing moderate grade (5–6%) downhill running, assisted bungee cord movement, and other "towing" mechanisms that aid in accelerating an athlete's movement.

E. Drills involving the athlete moving against increased horizontal or vertical load designed to improve stride length.

F. The distance covered with each stride.

13. _____ Multidirectional speed

14. _____ Quickness

15. _____ Total response time

16. _____ Reaction time

17. _____ Support phase

18. _____ Recovery phase

19. _____ Drive phase

G. The amount of time needed to complete a stride cycle.

H. The ability to move the body in one intended direction as fast as possible.

I. Where the foot contacts the ground well in front of the body's center of gravity.

J. A combination of foot/ankle plantar flexion, knee extension, and hip extension.

K. A combination of foot/ankle dorsiflexion, knee flexion, and hip flexion.

L. The ability to change direction or orientation of the body based on rapid processing of internal or external information quickly and accurately without significant loss of speed.

M. The ability to create speed in any direction or body orientation (forward, backward, lateral, diagonal).

N. An athlete's ability to execute movement skill in a comparatively brief amount of time.

O. The summation of the reaction time and the time it takes to execute the reactionary movement of concern.

P. When the foot is in contact with the ground.

Q. When the leg swings from the hip while the foot clears the ground.

R. Where the runner's weight is carried by the entire foot.

S. The time elapsed between the athlete's recognizing the need to act and initiating the appropriate action.

EXERCISE 9-2   True/False

1. Speed is a culmination of reactive ability, rapid force development, rapid force application, and effective movement technique.

   TRUE   FALSE

2. Speed cannot be trained or improved because it is strictly the result of genetics.

   TRUE   FALSE

3. Training the muscle and tendon's ability to load eccentrically and rapidly release energy concentrically improves the magnitude and effectiveness of the stretch-shortening cycle.

   TRUE   FALSE

4. If there is an imbalance of strength and flexibility about the hip, range of motion will be compromised, which will in turn affect force output and speed of movement.

   TRUE   FALSE

5. Overspeed/assisted drills are recommended for beginners and advanced athletes.

   TRUE   FALSE

6. Weight vests, sled pushes, and uphill running are examples of overspeed/assisted speed drills.

   TRUE   FALSE

7. During multidirectional movements, the body attempts to align itself as linearly as possible to maximize force production and running velocity.

   TRUE   FALSE

8. Research suggests that optimal stride length for maximal speed in sprinting is 1.3–1.5 times the athlete's leg length.

   TRUE   FALSE

9. The athlete who can apply speed, power, agility/multidirectional speed, and other game skills at the right time at the highest rate will be the most successful.

   TRUE   FALSE

10. Training for quickness is a process of taking all of the skills required for effective speed and agility in addition to the specific skills needed in a sport, and applying them to the reactionary demands of that sport.

    TRUE   FALSE

EXERCISE 9-3   Short Answer

INSTRUCTIONS: Briefly answer the following question.

1. Before designing programs to improve speed, agility/MDS, and quickness, what are the three most important aspects a Sports Performance Professional must address?

   _____

   _____

   _____

CHAPTER 10

Integrated Resistance Training for Performance Enhancement

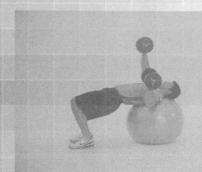

| | EXERCISE 10-1 | **Essential Vocabulary** |

PURPOSE: To gain an understanding of key terms used in Chapter 10 of the textbook.

INSTRUCTIONS: Match the terms with their proper definitions.

VOCABULARY WORDS

1. _____ Principle of individualization
2. _____ The principle of specificity (SAID Principle)
3. _____ Principle of overload
4. _____ General adaptation syndrome
5. _____ Exhaustion
6. _____ Alarm reaction
7. _____ Resistance development
8. _____ Periodization
9. _____ Hypertrophy
10. _____ Stabilization
11. _____ Mechanical specificity
12. _____ Neuromuscular specificity

DEFINITIONS

A. The principle that states that the body will undergo specific adaptations to the specific type of demand placed on it.

B. The principle that implies that there must be a training stimulus provided that exceeds the current capabilities of the kinetic chain to elicit the optimal physical, physiologic, and performance adaptations.

C. Refers to the uniqueness of a program to the client for whom it is designed.

D. A pattern of adaptation in which the kinetic chain responds and adapts to stressors to maintain homeostasis.

E. The initial reaction to a stressor.

F. When prolonged stress or stress that is intolerable to an athlete produces exhaustion or distress.

13. _____ Intermuscular coordination

14. _____ Intramuscular coordination

15. _____ Metabolic specificity

16. _____ Muscular endurance

17. _____ Power

18. _____ Strength

G. When the body increases its functional capacity to adapt to the stressor.

H. Division of a training program into smaller progressive stages.

I. The Human Movement System's ability to provide optimal dynamic joint support and maintain correct posture during all movements.

J. The enlargement of skeletal muscle fibers in response to being recruited to develop increased levels of tension.

K. Refers to the weight and movements placed on the body.

L. Refers to the speed of contraction and exercise selection.

M. Refers to the energy demand required for a specific activity.

N. The ability of the neuromuscular system to allow optimum levels of motor unit recruitment and motor unit synchronization within a single muscle using single joint exercises.

O. The ability of the neuromuscular system to allow all muscles to work together using multiple joint exercises.

P. The ability to produce and maintain force production over prolonged periods of time.

Q. The ability of the neuromuscular system to produce internal tension in order to overcome an external force.

R. The ability to generate the greatest possible force in the shortest amount of time.

EXERCISE 10-2   Multiple Choice

1. Which resistance training system uses one set for each exercise?

   a. Pyramid system
   b. Superset system
   c. Single-set system
   d. Split-routine system

2. Which resistance training system involves a step approach that either increases weight with each set or decreases weight with each set?

   a. Pyramid system
   b. Superset system
   c. Peripheral heart action system
   d. Circuit training system

3. Which resistance training system is another variation of circuit training that alternates upper-body and lower-body exercises throughout the circuit?

   a. Pyramid system
   b. Superset system
   c. Peripheral heart action system
   d. Split-routine system

4. Which of the following involves performing two exercises for antagonistic muscles?

   a. Pyramid system
   b. Peripheral heart action system
   c. Compound sets
   d. Trisets

5. Which resistance training system involves breaking the body up into parts to be trained on separate days?

   a. Pyramid system
   b. Peripheral heart action system
   c. Single-set system
   d. Split-routine system

6. Which resistance training system is used by NASM and follows the OPT™ model progressing a workout vertically down the template (total body → chest → back → shoulders → biceps → triceps → legs) in a circuit style minimizing rest periods in between exercises.

   a. Pyramid system
   b. Peripheral heart action system
   c. Vertical loading system
   d. Horizontal loading system

7. Which resistance training system requires performing all sets of an exercise or body part (with an adequate rest period between sets) before moving on to the next exercise or body part?

   a. Peripheral heart action system
   b. Circuit training system
   c. Horizontal loading system
   d. Vertical loading system

8. What is the PRIMARY goal of resistance-stabilization exercises?

   a. To improve neuromuscular efficiency, stability and prepares the neuromuscular system for the higher intensity activities to follow.
   b. To enhance prime mover strength allowing the athlete to handle heavier loads.
   c. To improve rate of force productions and overall muscular power.
   d. To improve anaerobic glycolysis capabilities.

9. What is the PRIMARY goal of resistance-strength exercises?

   a. To improve neuromuscular efficiency, stability and prepares the neuromuscular system for the higher intensity activities to follow.
   b. To enhance prime mover strength allowing the athlete to handle heavier loads.
   c. To improve rate of force productions and overall muscular power.
   d. To reduce aerobic oxidative capabilities.

10. What is the PRIMARY goal of resistance-power exercises?

   a. To improve neuromuscular efficiency, stability and prepares the neuromuscular system for the higher intensity activities to follow.
   b. To enhance prime mover strength allowing the athlete to handle heavier loads.
   c. To improve rate of force productions and overall muscular power.
   d. To reduce anaerobic glycolysis capabilities.

EXERCISE 10-3   **Matching**

INSTRUCTIONS: Answer the following questions referring to the images below.

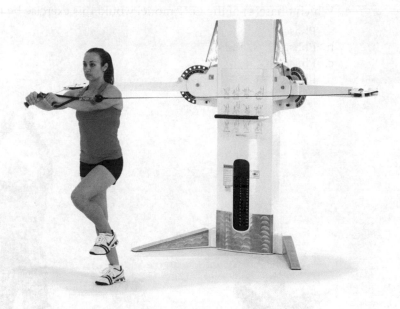

1. What type of chest exercise is illustrated above?
   a. Chest stabilization
   b. Chest strength
   c. Chest power

2. Which phase(s) of the OPT model would this exercise be most appropriate for?
   a. Phase 1
   b. Phases 2 and 3
   c. Phase 4
   d. Phases 5 and 6

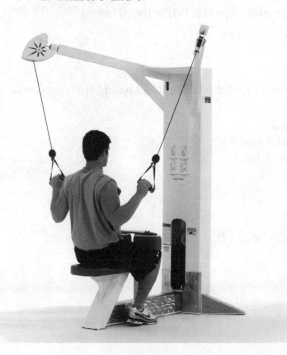

3. What type of back exercise is illustrated above?

    a. Back stabilization
    b. Back strength
    c. Back power

4. Which phase(s) of the OPT model would this exercise be most appropriate for?

    a. Phase 1
    b. Phases 2, 3, and 4
    c. Phase 5
    d. Phase 6

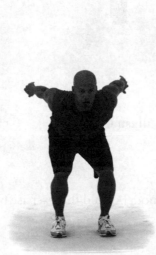

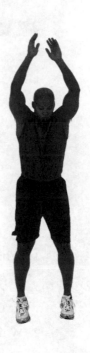

5. What type of leg exercise is illustrated above?

    a. Leg stabilization
    b. Leg strength
    c. Leg power

6. Which phase(s) of the OPT model would this exercise be most appropriate for?

    a. Phase 1
    b. Phase 2
    c. Phases 3 and 4
    d. Phases 5 and 6

CHAPTER 11

Olympic Lifting for Performance Enhancement

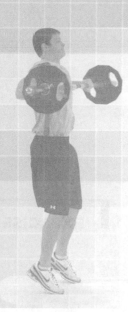

EXERCISE 11-1 Essential Vocabulary

PURPOSE: To gain an understanding of key terms used in Chapter 11 of the textbook.

INSTRUCTIONS: Match the terms with their proper definitions.

VOCABULARY WORDS

1. _____ Rate of force development

2. _____ High-load speed strength

3. _____ Maximum strength

4. _____ Skill performance

5. _____ Reactive strength

6. _____ Power endurance

7. _____ Hip hinge

8. _____ Neutral spine

9. _____ Work capacity

10. _____ Perturbation

DEFINITIONS

A. According to the force-velocity curve, the highest forces are generated at slow contraction velocities.

B. The greatest amount of force generated, typically measured during a 1 RM.

C. The time the mechanical, electrical, and elastic properties of the neuromuscular system respond to a stimulus to reach the required force.

D. The necessary strength in response to some sort of stimulus, be it physical, visual, or auditory.

E. The learning of a new skill whereby unnecessary motor units are eliminated and the skill progressively becomes relegated to almost a subconscious level.

F. The ability to sustain a high-power output for an extended period of time.

G. A posture where there is no exaggeration of any of the normal curvatures of the spine.

H. The spine remaining stiff and neutral while movement occurs about the hip joint.

I. Any disruption in the normal pattern of movement; a disturbance in the relationship of the center of mass to the base of support.

J. The maximum amount of work that a person can handle and will vary based on the intensity-duration relationship of the task.

EXERCISE 11-2   True/False

1. The competition lifts of Olympic weightlifting are the snatch and the clean & jerk.
   TRUE   FALSE

2. Derivatives of the Olympic lifts include the power snatch, power clean, snatch and clean pulls, squats, and deadlifts.
   TRUE   FALSE

3. The second pull phase of the snatch and power snatch exhibit the highest-power outputs of any resistance training exercise.
   TRUE   FALSE

4. According to research, Olympic lifts do not improve vertical jump performance.
   TRUE   FALSE

5. The power clean and power snatch require greater dorsiflexion and hip flexion when compared to the snatch and clean & jerk used in competition.
   TRUE   FALSE

6. A limited range of shoulder flexion due to tightness in the latissimus dorsi can lead to excessive lumbar extension.
   TRUE   FALSE

7. As the athlete learns how to stabilize the trunk and can perform the lifting techniques properly, load can then be increased allowing for greater strength gains of both the local and global systems of the core.
   TRUE   FALSE

8. The athlete who is unable to achieve the posture necessary to lift a weight from the floor should have his or her starting position changed with the use of blocks combined with flexibility and stability exercises to improve postural control.
   TRUE   FALSE

9. If torso and core stability is poor or nonexistent, then the gluteus maximus may not fire with the proper timing and intensity as the primary hip extensor leading to synergistic dominance of the lumbar extensors and hamstrings.
   TRUE   FALSE

10. If compensations are present when performing the overhead and single-leg squat assessments, Olympic lifting may not be a viable option until movement deficiencies are corrected.
    TRUE   FALSE

EXERCISE 11-3   Multiple Choice

1. Which exercise is sometimes described as a single movement as the weight is pulled from the floor with two hands and explosively lifted to arm's length over the head with no pause in the movement?

   a. Clean & jerk
   b. Snatch
   c. Power clean
   d. Back squat

2. When performing the snatch, the first pull phase occurs when

   a. the barbell is lifted from the floor to knee height.
   b. the barbell is elevated from the knees to an area between the mid-thigh and the pubic bone.
   c. a violent extension of the hips, knees, and ankles helps drive the bar upward and slightly forward off the upper thigh or pubic area.
   d. lifter drops rapidly into a squat position, moving the feet quickly sideways and extending the arms overhead to catch the bar.

3. Which lifting exercise enables athletes to achieve the heaviest weights overhead?

   a. Snatch
   b. Power snatch
   c. Clean & jerk
   d. Power clean

4. Which lifting exercise requires the widest grip?

   a. Snatch
   b. Clean & jerk
   c. Hang clean
   d. Power clean

5. The tendency of the barbell to move forward and away from the body during the first pull should be counteracted by the isometric contraction of the:

   a. latissimus dorsi
   b. gastrocnemius
   c. biceps femoris
   d. upper trapezius

6. Place the phases of the snatch exercise in the correct order.

   a. Getting set → the shift (scoop) → first pull → top pull → the amortization (catch)
   b. Getting set → first pull → the shift (scoop) → top pull → the amortization (catch)
   c. Getting set → the shift (scoop) → the amortization (catch) → top pull → first pull
   d. Getting set → the shift (scoop) → first pull → the amortization (catch) → top pull

7. Which exercise is a good alternative to the clean when the full squat position cannot be achieved?

   a. Snatch
   b. Power clean
   c. Clean & jerk
   d. Barbell overhead squat

8. All of the following are stability cues to improve core stabilization and proper exercise technique EXCEPT

   a. drawing-in.
   b. abdominal bracing.
   c. scapular retraction.
   d. anterior pelvic tilt.

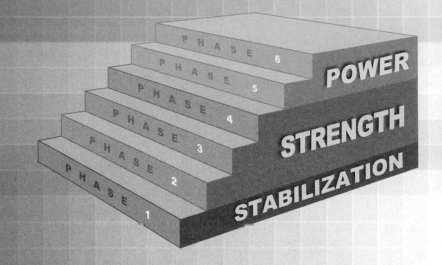

SECTION 4

Program Design
Principles and
Application

CHAPTER 12

The Science of Periodization and the Optimum Performance Training™ Model

EXERCISE 12-1 Essential Vocabulary

PURPOSE: To gain an understanding of key terms used in Chapter 12 of the textbook.

INSTRUCTIONS: Match the terms with their proper definitions.

VOCABULARY WORDS

1. _____ Training duration
2. _____ Training frequency
3. _____ Acute variables
4. _____ Training volume
5. _____ Training intensity
6. _____ Repetition tempo
7. _____ Rest interval
8. _____ Exercise selection
9. _____ Undulating periodization
10. _____ Corrective exercise training

DEFINITIONS

A. Important components that specify how each exercise is to be performed.

B. An individual's level of effort, compared to their maximal effort, which is usually expressed as a percentage.

C. The speed with which each repetition is performed.

D. The time taken to recuperate between sets.

E. Amount of physical training performed within a specified time period.

F. The process of choosing appropriate exercises for a client's program.

G. Training at varying intensities during the course of a week, which allows for multiple adaptations once a level of fitness has been achieved.

H. Designed to correct muscle imbalances, joint dysfunctions, neuromuscular deficits, and postural distortion patterns that the athlete may have developed during the season.

I. The time frame of a workout or the length of time spent in one phase of training.

J. The number of training sessions performed over a specified time period (usually 1 week).

EXERCISE 12-2   True/False

1. The best way to achieve consistent, superior results is to follow a periodized training program.
   TRUE   FALSE

2. Acute variables are the most fundamental components of designing a training program because they determine the amount of stress placed upon the body and, ultimately, what adaptation the body will incur.
   TRUE   FALSE

3. The number of repetitions performed in a given set is dependent upon the athlete's work capacity, intensity of the exercise, and the specific phase of training.
   TRUE   FALSE

4. Power adaptations require 1–10 repetitions at 30–45% of the one-repetition maximum (1RM) or approximately 10% of body weight.
   TRUE   FALSE

5. Endurance is BEST achieved by performing 8–12 repetitions at 70–85% of the 1RM.
   TRUE   FALSE

6. Hypertrophy is BEST achieved utilizing 8–12 repetitions at 70–85% of the 1RM.
   TRUE   FALSE

7. If maximal strength adaptations are desired, the desired repetition range is 1–10 at 30–45% of the 1RM.
   TRUE   FALSE

8. Research demonstrates that approximately 25–40% of a traditional "Explosive Power" lift requires deceleration.
   TRUE   FALSE

9. Corrective exercise training is designed to correct muscle imbalances, joint dysfunctions, neuromuscular deficits, and postural distortion patterns that the athlete may have developed during the season.
   TRUE   FALSE

10. A mesocycle is the largest cycle and typically covers a yearlong period of training (the annual plan).
    TRUE   FALSE

EXERCISE 12-3   Multiple Choice

1. All of the following are PRIMARY goals/adaptations of Phase 1 Stabilization Endurance EXCEPT
   a. increase in stability.
   b. increase in muscular endurance.
   c. increasing neuromuscular efficiency of the core musculature.
   d. increased muscular development (hypertrophy).

2. Which phase of the OPT™ model entails the use of superset techniques in which a more stable exercise (such as a bench press) is immediately followed with a stabilization exercise with similar biomechanical motions (such as a stability ball push-up)?
   a. Phase 1 Stabilization Endurance training
   b. Phase 2 Strength Endurance training

    c. Phase 3 Hypertrophy training
    d. Phase 4 Maximal Strength training

3. Which phase of the OPT model is specific for the adaptation of maximal muscle growth, focusing on high levels of volume with minimal rest periods to force cellular changes that result in an overall increase in muscle size?

    a. Phase 1 Stabilization Endurance training
    b. Phase 2 Strength Endurance training
    c. Phase 3 Hypertrophy training
    d. Phase 4 Maximal Strength training

4. All of the following are PRIMARY adaptations of Phase 4 Maximal Strength training EXCEPT

    a. increase in recruitment of motor units.
    b. increase in rate of force production.
    c. increase in motor unit synchronization.
    d. increase in muscular endurance.

5. Which phase of the OPT model utilizes a form of complex training, supersetting a strength exercise with a power exercise for each body part?

    a. Phase 3 Hypertrophy training
    b. Phase 4 Maximal Strength training
    c. Phase 5 Power training
    d. Phase 6 Maximal Power training

6. What is the PRIMARY focus of Phase 6 Maximal Power training?

    a. Increase in stability
    b. Increased in muscular development (hypertrophy)
    c. Increasing maximal strength
    d. Increase in velocity (speed)

7. Which phase of the OPT model utilizes 1–5 repetitions at 85–100% of 1RM during resistance exercises?

    a. Phase 3 Hypertrophy training
    b. Phase 4 Maximal Strength training
    c. Phase 5 Power training
    d. Phase 6 Maximal Power training

8. A rest interval of 20–30 seconds replenishes what percentage of ATP/CP stores?

    a. 10
    b. 30
    c. 50
    d. 90

9. Volume is inversely related to what?

    a. Goals
    b. General fitness level
    c. Recoverability
    d. Intensity

10. Which phase of the OPT model primarily progresses exercises by increasing the proprioceptive demand (controlled instability) rather than the load?

    a. Phase 1 Stabilization Endurance training
    b. Phase 2 Strength Endurance training
    c. Phase 3 Hypertrophy training
    d. Phase 4 Maximal Strength training

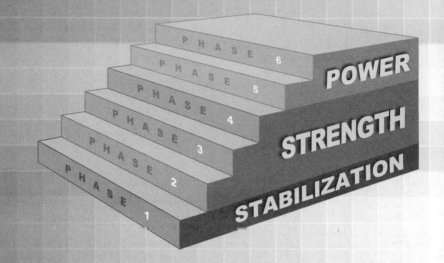

SECTION 5

Injury Prevention
and Reconditioning

CHAPTER 13

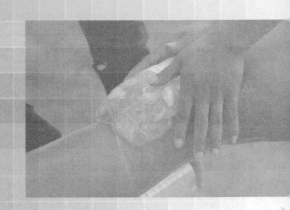

Current Concepts in Injury Prevention and Reconditioning

▌ EXERCISE 13-1 Essential Vocabulary

PURPOSE: To gain an understanding of key terms used in Chapter 13 of the textbook.

INSTRUCTIONS: Match the terms with their proper definitions.

VOCABULARY WORDS

1. _____ Q-angle

2. _____ Plantar fascia

3. _____ High ankle sprain

4. _____ Subacromial impingement syndrome (SAIS)

5. _____ Metatarsal stress fracture

6. _____ Patellofemoral pain

7. _____ Achilles tendonitis

8. _____ Anterior cruciate ligament (ACL)

DEFINITIONS

A. A thick, fibrous band of tissue that runs from the calcaneus and fans out to insert on the metatarsal heads to support the longitudinal arch of the foot.

B. Fractures occurring to the long bones of the foot between the phalanges and the tarsals.

C. Inflammation to the tendon shared by the gastrocnemius and soleus muscles that inserts on the base of the calcaneus.

D. A syndesmotic sprain involving the distal tibiofibular joint just proximal to the ankle.

E. A symptom that is provoked or accentuated by action that involve motion at the patellofemoral joint and/or increase pressure of the patella against the femoral condyles

F. Primary stabilizing ligament of the knee whose primary function is to prevent anterior displacement of the tibia relative to the femur.

G. A line drawn from the anterior superior iliac spine to the central patella and a second line drawn from central patella through the tibial tubercle.

H. Compression of the structures that run beneath the coracoacromial arch, most often from a decrease in the subacromial space.

EXERCISE 13-2   True/False

1. Some common mechanisms of Achilles tendonitis include overuse, poorly fitted shoes, and eccentric loading.
   TRUE   FALSE

2. Plantar fasciitis is PRIMARILY an overuse syndrome.
   TRUE   FALSE

3. The most common metatarsal stress fractures occur to the second and fifth metatarsals.
   TRUE   FALSE

4. Ankle sprains are reported to be the most common sports-related injury, and the No. 1 injury for time lost.
   TRUE   FALSE

5. Medial ankle sprains are far more common than lateral and high ankle sprains.
   TRUE   FALSE

6. The typical mechanism of injury for a lateral ankle sprain is forced dorsiflexion and eversion of the ankle during landing.
   TRUE   FALSE

7. The most common risk factor for lateral ankle sprain is a history of a prior sprain.
   TRUE   FALSE

8. The most common mechanism of injury for a medial ankle sprain involves forceful and rapid inversion of the foot.
   TRUE   FALSE

9. The proposed mechanism of injury for high ankle sprains includes external foot rotation, talar eversion in the ankle mortise, and excessive dorsiflexion.
   TRUE   FALSE

10. One of the most commonly accepted causes of patellofemoral pain syndrome is abnormal tracking of the patella within the femoral trochlea.
    TRUE   FALSE

11. ACL injuries are overwhelmingly (70–75%) noncontact in nature and almost always occur as the body undergoes rapid deceleration.
    TRUE   FALSE

12. Researchers have suggested that the oblique fibers of the vastus medialis must activate earlier or at the same time as the vastus lateralis because a delay in vastus medialis oblique activation may lateralize the patella, leading to suboptimal tracking and increased stress on the patellar surface, cartilage damage, and pain.
    TRUE   FALSE

13. A large Q-angle is believed to facilitate excessive medial tracking of the patella.

    TRUE   FALSE

14. Femoral adduction has been proposed to cause an increase in the knee valgus angle and, in turn, lateral tracking of the patella.

    TRUE   FALSE

15. Specific movement patterns commonly occurring during ACL and lower-extremity injury include knee valgus (knock knee), excessive leg rotation, and decreased knee flexion.

    TRUE   FALSE

16. Proprioception-balance training and plyometric-agility training shown to successfully alter movement patterns by decreasing visible knee valgus, minimizing tibial rotation, and increasing knee flexion angle are instrumental in reducing the incidence of knee injury during sport and recreational activities.

    TRUE   FALSE

▌ EXERCISE 13-3   Multiple Choice

1. Some common risk factors for plantar fasciitis include all of the following EXCEPT
   a. less than 0 degree ankle dorsiflexion.
   b. body mass index greater than 30.
   c. increased foot pronation.
   d. 20 degrees of ankle dorsiflexion.

2. Which local muscles have diminished activation in patients with low-back pain?
   a. Transverse abdominus, multifidus
   b. Rectus abdominus, rectus femoris
   c. Psoas major, tensor fascia latae
   d. Adductor magnus, adductor brevis

3. Contraction of the _____ _____ is more effective at increasing SIJ stability than the larger abdominal muscles like the rectus abdominus and external oblique.
   a. psoas major
   b. rectus femoris
   c. serratus anterior
   d. transverse abdominus

4. A low-back injury prevention program should include a variety of exercises aimed at increasing all of the following EXCEPT
   a. flexibility of tight (overactive) muscles.
   b. strengthening weak (inhibited) muscles.
   c. neuromuscular control.
   d. synergistic dominance.

5. All of the following are corrective/injury prevention strategies for shoulder impairment EXCEPT
   a. soft tissue mobilization and self-myofascial release techniques to increase extensibility of overactive muscles.
   b. static or neuromuscular stretching of overactive muscles.
   c. isolated strengthening exercises to facilitate the underactive muscles of the scapulae.
   d. isolated strengthening exercises for overactive muscles.

6. SAIS involves all the following impinged structures EXCEPT
   a. supraspinatus tendon.
   b. infraspinatus tendon.
   c. Achilles tendon.
   d. long head of the biceps tendon.

7. SAIS may be the result of all of the following EXCEPT
   a. bony deformity of the acromion.
   b. scapular retraction and depression.
   c. shoulder instability.
   d. rotator cuff weakness.

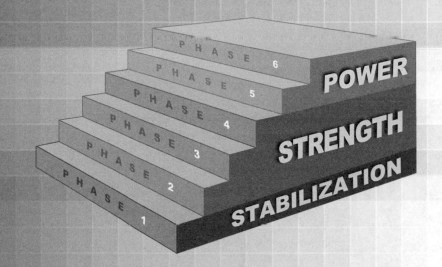

SECTION 6

Sports Nutrition and Performance Aids

CHAPTER 14

Performance Nutrition

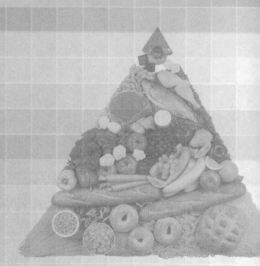

EXERCISE 14-1   **Essential Vocabulary**

PURPOSE: To gain an understanding of key terms used in Chapter 14 of the textbook.

INSTRUCTIONS: Match the terms with their proper definitions.

VOCABULARY WORDS

1. _____ Casein

2. _____ Dietetics

3. _____ Gluconeogenesis

4. _____ Glycemic index

5. _____ Performance nutrition

6. _____ Female athlete triad

7. _____ Hyponatremia

8. _____ Eicosanoid

DEFINITIONS

A. A combination of strategies to enhance physical and athletic performance through specific food and nutrient choices, timing, and quantities.

B. A "slow" protein because of its moderate, prolonged amino acid increase.

C. The practice of nutrition governed by national credentialing programs and state licensing laws.

D. A ranking system of carbohydrate foods indicating the effect on circulating blood glucose and insulin levels.

E. A metabolic pathway that results in the generation of glucose from noncarbohydrate carbon substrates such as pyruvate, lactate, glycerol, and glucogenic amino acids.

F. A combination of an eating disorder, amenorrhea, and osteoporosis (low bone mass) often experienced by female athletes.

G. Signaling molecules made by oxygenation of 20-carbon essential fatty acids. They exert complex control over many bodily systems, mainly in inflammation or immunity, and as messengers in the central nervous system.

H. An electrolyte disturbance in which the sodium concentration in the plasma is too low (below 135 mmol/L).

▌ EXERCISE 14-2   True/False

1. Providing individual nutrition assessment, dietary advice, meal plans, and recommendations for supplements or nutrient intakes is well within the scope of practice for a Sports Performance Professional.

   TRUE   FALSE

2. At 65% or more of $\dot{V}O_2$max, carbohydrate is the body's predominant fuel.

   TRUE   FALSE

3. Generally, the greater the preexercise glycogen stores, the longer an athlete can exercise.

   TRUE   FALSE

4. In the postexercise period, an athlete wants to ingest carbohydrates that are digested and absorbed slowly (low gastrointestinal) to help enhance muscle recovery and glycogen repletion.

   TRUE   FALSE

5. Carbohydrate loading can almost double muscle glycogen concentrations, which can ultimately impact endurance potential and is most effective for athletes performing intense, continuous endurance activities lasting longer than 90 minutes.

   TRUE   FALSE

6. Athletes have increased requirements of protein because of the need to repair exercise-related muscle damage, support lean mass gains, and replace proteins used as energy.

   TRUE   FALSE

7. Strength and power athletes consuming more than 1.6–1.7 g/kg of body mass per day has not been proven to be any more effective at increasing lean mass.

   TRUE   FALSE

8. The need for protein may be lower during the first 3–6 months of training when muscle hypertrophy rates are accelerated.

   TRUE   FALSE

9. Fat helps athletes meet daily calorie needs, maintain body temperature, protect organs, deliver and absorb fat-soluble vitamins and carotenoids, enhance taste and texture of foods, and improve the satiety of meals and snacks.

   TRUE   FALSE

10. Very low-fat diets (<15% of total calories as fat) compared with moderate fat diets (20–25% of total calories as fat) have shown no performance benefit.

   TRUE   FALSE

EXERCISE 14-3   Multiple Choice

1. The greatest risk for micronutrient deficiencies includes all of the following EXCEPT

   a. restricting calorie intake.
   b. eliminating one or more foods groups from an athlete's daily diet.
   c. consuming high-calorie, low-nutrient dense diets.
   d. consuming 25 g of fiber per day.

2. How much protein is recommended for strength and power athletes consume?

   a. 1.6–1.7 g/kg
   b. 0.8–0.9 g/kg
   c. 0.4–0.5 g/kg
   d. 0.2–0.3 g/kg

3. How much protein is generally recommended for endurance athletes?

   a. 0.2–0.4 g/kg
   b. 0.5–0.7 g/kg
   c. 0.8–1.0 g/kg
   d. 1.2–1.4 g/kg

4. What is the acceptable macronutrient distribution range of fat intake for all adults?

   a. 0–5% of daily energy intake
   b. 10–15% of daily energy intake
   c. 20–35% of daily energy intake
   d. 40–50% of daily energy intake

5. Which micronutrient may help reduce muscle soreness and damage induced by exercise-associated oxidative stress and may help reduce upper respiratory tract infection duration?

   a. Iron
   b. Vitamin C
   c. Folate
   d. Calcium

6. Consuming a pre-event or pre-exercise meal should utilize all of the following guidelines EXCEPT

   a. sufficient fluids to maintain hydration.
   b. low in fat and fiber to encourage gastric emptying and minimize gastrointestinal distress.
   c. high in carbohydrate to optimize glycogen stores.
   d. little or no protein.

7. The key to maximizing recovery is to consume high glycemic carbohydrates and proteins in a 4:1 ratio within

   a. 30–45 minutes after exercise.
   b. 60 minutes after exercise.
   c. 90 minutes after exercise.
   d. 2 hours after exercise.

8. A failure to meet energy needs leads to all of the following EXCEPT

   a. decreases in performance.
   b. decreased immune and reproductive function.
   c. reduction in weight.
   d. increase in lean body mass and fat mass.

9. A positive net protein balance is BEST achieved through the use of the following strategies EXCEPT

   a. consume a mixture of carbohydrate and amino acids before and immediately after strength workouts.
   b. adequately replenish glycogen stores immediately after workouts.
   c. meet daily carbohydrate needs.
   d. consuming a high-protein low-carbohydrate diet.

10. What is the 2004 dietary reference intakes recommendation for adequate water for males and females?

   a. 80 oz/day (10 cups) for males and 64 oz/day (8 cups) for females
   b. 130 oz/day for males (16 cups) and 95 oz/day (12 cups) for females
   c. 200 oz/day for males (25 cups) and 150 oz/day (19 cups) for females
   d. 240 oz/day for males (30 cups) and 195 oz/day (24 cups) for females

CHAPTER 15

Ergogenic Aids

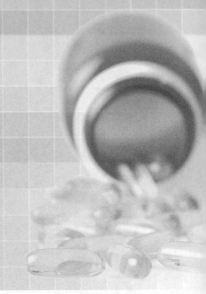

EXERCISE 15-1 Essential Vocabulary

PURPOSE: To gain an understanding of key terms used in Chapter 15 of the textbook.

INSTRUCTIONS: Match the terms with their proper definitions.

VOCABULARY WORDS

1. _____ Ergolytic

2. _____ Central fatigue

3. _____ Ergogenic

4. _____ Nonanemic iron deficiency

5. _____ Anticatabolic substances

6. _____ Blood doping

7. _____ Androgenic anabolic steroids

8. _____ Serotonin

9. _____ Amenorrheic athletes

DEFINITIONS

A. Literally means "work generating"

B. Impaired performance

C. Increased brain levels of the neuro-transmitter serotonin causing the sensation of tiredness and fatigue.

D. A state in which iron reserves have been depleted and the body is drawing on limited tissue sources of iron to maintain red blood cell production.

E. Substances thought to reduce muscle protein catabolism (breakdown) by protecting muscle protein and promoting building and maintaining muscle mass.

F. Drugs designed to mimic the effects of testosterone promoting the building of muscle mass, strength, and loss of body fat, but at the risk of serious adverse health effects.

G. A practice that can increase maximal oxygen uptake and enhance endurance performance by removing blood from an athlete and storing the red blood cells in a frozen form until red blood cells (in a saline solution) are infused back into the athlete at a later date.

H. Female athletes with the absence of a menstrual period during reproductive ages.

I. A neurotransmitter in the modulation of anger, aggression, body temperature, mood, sleep, sexuality, appetite, and metabolism.

EXERCISE 15-2   True/False

1. An effective physiological, pharmacological, or nutritional ergogenic aid generally enhances the body's ability to perform specific types of biochemical or physiological functions that are highly involved in supporting specific types of sports performance.

   TRUE   FALSE

2. A single, acute ingestion of creatine is unlikely to have any significant effects on exercise performance.

   TRUE   FALSE

3. Once a nutrient deficiency is corrected, consuming more than an adequate intake of that essential nutrient is unlikely to further enhance performance.

   TRUE   FALSE

4. Adequate and properly timed intake of water, carbohydrate, protein, and fat is the foundation for meeting the physiological demands of a particular sport.

   TRUE   FALSE

5. Dehydration is thought to occur when roughly 0.5% of body weight is lost because of sweat loss during exercise.

   TRUE   FALSE

6. Nutritional planning that matches the demands of a particular sport may be the best ergogenic aid available to athletes.

   TRUE   FALSE

7. Iron supplementation can have ergogenic effects in someone with poor iron status but could seriously impair performance and health in someone with the genetic condition of hemochromatosis (iron overload predisposition) if their iron stores are already high.

   TRUE   FALSE

8. Although excessive intake of some vitamins can seriously damage health, moderate supplementation likely is safe with the possible exception of vitamin A.

   TRUE   FALSE

9. Iron is one of the minerals most likely to be deficient in athletes, especially females, and iron deficiency anemia reduces the capacity for physical exertion.

   TRUE   FALSE

EXERCISE 15-3 Multiple Choice

1. The _____ _____ _____ proposes that increased brain levels of the neurotransmitter serotonin may cause the sensation of tiredness and fatigue.

   a. Central Fatigue Hypothesis
   b. Law of Energy
   c. Law of Thermodynamics
   d. Plummer-Vinson Syndrome

2. All of the following are potential adverse effects of androgenic-anabolic steroid use EXCEPT

   a. acne.
   b. loss of head hair.
   c. mental acuity.
   d. altered libido.

3. Amenorrheic athletes should automatically increase _____ intakes to a minimum of 1,500 mg/day.

   a. dehydroepiandrosterone
   b. androstenedione
   c. creatine
   d. calcium

4. Which of the following is produced naturally in the body and can serve as a precursor for androstenedione that, in turn, can be converted into testosterone or estrogens?

   a. Glutamine
   b. Adenosine triphosphate
   c. Dehydroepiandrosterone
   d. Tryptophan

5. Daily iron needs are _____ times higher for vegetarians because the iron in most plant foods is not absorbed as efficiently as it is from animal foods.

   a. 0.2
   b. 0.6
   c. 1.0
   d. 1.8

6. Which is NOT a potential negative effect of caffeine supplementation?

   a. Insomnia
   b. Nausea
   c. Rapid heart and breathing rates
   d. Energy for high-intensity short-duration activities

7. Which supplementation is not banned by a majority of major sports governing bodies?

   a. Blood doping
   b. Androgenic anabolic steroids
   c. Creatine
   d. Androstenedione

8. All of the following are inherent risks of blood doping EXCEPT

   a. contracting blood-borne diseases.
   b. bacterial infections.
   c. greater resistance to blood flow (sluggish blood).
   d. decreased maximal oxygen uptake.

9. Which of the following is a popular prohormone unlikely to be ergogenic for any athlete in normal health and is clearly not worth its potential downsides.
   a. Multivitamin
   b. Creatine
   c. Androstenedione
   d. Calcium

10. _____ is known to enhance the synthesis of growth hormone and insulin, benefit immune regulation, and stimulate dilation of blood vessels via nitric oxide synthesis; however, the limited research conducted to date does not support its effects on sports performance.
    a. Arginine
    b. Glycogen
    c. Creatine
    d. Triglycerides

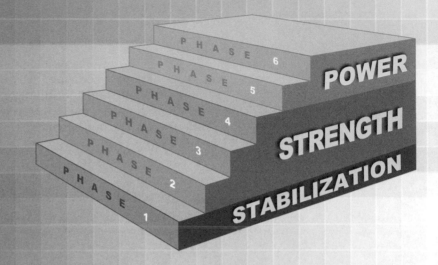

SECTION 7

Sports Psychology

CHAPTER 16

Performance Psychology: Integrating Physical and Mental Training

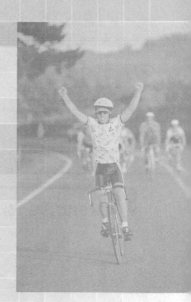

EXERCISE 16-1 Essential Vocabulary

PURPOSE: To gain an understanding of key terms used in Chapter 16 of the textbook.

INSTRUCTIONS: Match the terms with their proper definitions.

VOCABULARY WORDS

1. _____ Flow

2. _____ Self-talk

3. _____ Fight or flight

DEFINITIONS

A. A state of consciousness where one becomes totally absorbed in what one is doing to the exclusion of all other thoughts and emotions.

B. A physiological response stating that animals/humans react to threats with a general discharge of the sympathetic nervous system, priming the animal/human for fighting or fleeing.

C. The inner and outer dialog that forms our thoughts and shared ideas.

EXERCISE 16-2 Short Answer

INSTRUCTIONS: Briefly answer the following questions.

1. Describe the concept of "no-mind" or more commonly referred to as the "zone" in the athletic community.

_____

_____

_____

2. What are some appropriate questions to determine how an athlete (client) previously reached an "ideal mindset"?

_____

_____

_____

3. Why is it important to reengage the athlete's ideal mindset by asking questions that direct focus to the present moment?

_____

_____

_____

EXERCISE 16-3   True/False

1. According to Csikszentmihalyi, "flow" is more likely to occur in moments when the demands of the situation are challenging and the athlete perceives his or her skills to be sufficient to meet those demands.
   TRUE   FALSE

2. If challenges are perceived to be too low, boredom is the likely result.
   TRUE   FALSE

3. Experts in sport psychology have reported that the ability to focus on task-relevant cues is a necessary ingredient for performance success.
   TRUE   FALSE

4. In regards to sport performance, the more one focuses on the environment, the more slowly time seems to pass.
   TRUE   FALSE

5. The Sports Performance Professional can assist in slowing down the game by training athletes to focus their attention internally (thoughts, feelings, or internal images) during critical and decisive moments in training.
   TRUE   FALSE

6. The "fight or flight" mechanism results in physiological reactions including muscle relaxation, decreased respiration rate, and decreased heart rate.
   TRUE   FALSE

7. The perception of the inability to cope may lead to a less optimal emotional state and subsequent performance decrements.
   TRUE   FALSE

8. Effective goal setting has been linked to performance enhancement.
   TRUE   FALSE

9. Some factors that negatively impact confidence include negative self-talk, a narrowing of attention on performance mistakes, and fixation with the skill level of the opponent.
   TRUE   FALSE

10. Some tools to manage over-intensity include self-talk, familiarization with the competitive arena, having contingency plans, controlling the controllable, breathing, centering, muscle relaxation, imagery, cue words, pre-performance routines, smiling, laughter, and music.
    TRUE   FALSE

APPENDIX

Answers to Exercises

Chapter 1

EXERCISE 1-1

1. G	4. F	6. D
2. C	5. E	7. A
3. B		

EXERCISE 1-2

Integrated training is a comprehensive approach that attempts to improve all components necessary for an athlete to perform at the highest level and prevent injury. Integrated training does this by focusing on developing *functional strength* and *neuromuscular efficiency*.

EXERCISE 1-3

1. True	5. True	8. True
2. True	6. True	9. True
3. True	7. False	10. False
4. True		

Chapter 2

EXERCISE 2-1

1. E	7. B	12. J
2. G	8. M	13. N
3. A	9. L	14. F
4. D	10. O	15. I
5. C	11. K	16. P
6. H		

EXERCISE 2-2

1. Sagittal plane	4. Pronation	7. Isometric contraction
2. Frontal plane	5. Supination	8. Concentric contraction
3. Transverse plane	6. Eccentric contraction	

EXERCISE 2-3

1. a	4. d	6. c
2. b	5. a	7. d
3. c		

Chapter 3

EXERCISE 3-1

1. D
2. A
3. B
4. C

EXERCISE 3-2

1. True
2. True
3. True
4. True
5. True
6. False
7. True
8. False
9. True
10. False

EXERCISE 3-3

1. a
2. b
3. d
4. a
5. c
6. c
7. d
8. a
9. b
10. c
11. c
12. d

EXERCISE 3-4

1. b
2. c
3. a
4. d
5. a
6. d
7. a
8. b
9. a
10. d
11. d
12. a

Chapter 4

EXERCISE 4-1

1. C
2. H
3. F
4. A
5. B
6. D
7. E
8. G
9. J
10. N
11. I
12. K
13. L
14. M

EXERCISE 4-2

1. True
2. False
3. True
4. True
5. True
6. False
7. True
8. True
9. True
10. True

EXERCISE 4-3

Muscle imbalances can be caused by problems ranging from postural stress to decreased recovery and delayed regeneration. Some additional causes of muscle imbalances include pattern overload, poor technical skill, aging, lack of core strength, immobilization, cumulative trauma, and lack of neuromuscular control. These muscle imbalances result in altered reciprocal inhibition, synergistic dominance, arthrokinetic dysfunction, and decreased neuromuscular control.

EXERCISE 4-4

1. b	5. b	8. a
2. a	6. d	9. b
3. c	7. c	10. a
4. a		

Chapter 5

EXERCISE 5-1

1. E	5. B	8. F
2. G	6. C	9. I
3. A	7. D	10. J
4. H		

EXERCISE 5-2

1. True	5. True	8. True
2. True	6. False	9. False
3. True	7. False	10. False
4. True		

EXERCISE 5-3

1. During a Phase 1 Base Training program, the athlete will have a low-intensity day (Zone 1 or 65–75% of HRMax) and a higher-intensity day in which the athlete will be slowly introduced to Zone 2 (80–85% of HRMax). This creates a 2-day rotation. Day 1 consists of a cardiorespiratory workout in Zone 1. Day 2 consists of an interval workout flip-flopping between Zone 1 and Zone 2.

2. Phase 2 Interval Training creates a 3-day rotation, 1 day for each training zone. Day 1 is a low-intensity day in Zone 1, acting as a recovery day from the higher-intensity days. In day 2, the athlete spends the majority of the workout in Zone 2. Day 3 is the true interval day. For example, the athlete performs three 1-minute sprints in Zones 2 and 3 inside of a 5-minute interval followed by a true recovery in Zone 1.

3. Phases 3 through 5 of the cardio programming focus on outdoor drills that help improve conditioning through the use of linear and multidirectional sprints as well as using sport-specific drills performed as conditioning practice.
   - Phase 3 Linear Training
   - Phase 4 Multidirectional Training
   - Phase 5 Sport Specific Training

4. Signs and symptoms of overtraining include
   - the inability to reach training zones.
   - inadequate sleep at night.
   - workouts that are described by the client as "draining"
   - a client's lack of feeling "refreshed" at the end of the workout.

Chapter 6

EXERCISE 6-1

1. D	5. C	8. I
2. G	6. E	9. H
3. A	7. F	10. J
4. B		

EXERCISE 6-2

1. a	3. b	5. c
2. a	4. b	6. d

EXERCISE 6-3

1. True	5. True	8. False
2. True	6. False	9. True
3. True	7. True	10. True
4. False		

Chapter 7

EXERCISE 7-1

1. C	5. A	9. J
2. D	6. G	10. K
3. B	7. F	11. I
4. E	8. H	

EXERCISE 7-2

1. True	5. False	8. False
2. True	6. True	9. False
3. True	7. False	10. True
4. True		

EXERCISE 7-3

1. Sports Performance Professionals must understand postural control and its components to efficiently and effectively train athletes to achieve optimum performance. The apparently simple act of maintaining an athletic position during sport is actually a continuing process of minute adjustments to keep the athlete's center of gravity over their base of support. The smaller the base of support (e.g., on a single leg) the more precise and accurate the postural adjustments need to be to keep the center of gravity over the base of support.

    Research has demonstrated that balance training restores dynamic stabilization mechanisms, improves neuromuscular efficiency, and stimulates joint and muscle receptors to encourage maximal sensory input to the central nervous system. Acting collectively, this improves proprioception, kinesthesia, and neuromuscular efficiency (central processing), which in turn can improve performance and decrease injury.

EXERCISE 7-4

1. c	3. a	5. b
2. d	4. a	6. b

Chapter 8

EXERCISE 8-1

1. A	3. E	5. F
2. B	4. D	6. C

EXERCISE 8-2

1. True	4. False	6. True
2. True	5. False	7. False
3. True		

EXERCISE 8-3

1. b	5. d	9. b
2. a	6. a	10. c
3. c	7. a	11. d
4. a	8. b	

Chapter 9

EXERCISE 9-1

1. D	8. F	14. N
2. C	9. I	15. O
3. A	10. K	16. S
4. B	11. J	17. R
5. E	12. L	18. Q
6. H	13. M	19. P
7. G		

EXERCISE 9-2

1. True	5. False	8. False
2. False	6. False	9. True
3. True	7. True	10. True
4. True		

EXERCISE 9-3

1. When designing programs to improve SAQ, the needs of the athlete, the needs of the specific sport, and proper organization and integration should be addressed.

Chapter 10

EXERCISE 10-1

1. C	7. G	13. O
2. A	8. H	14. N
3. B	9. J	15. M
4. D	10. I	16. P
5. F	11. K	17. R
6. E	12. L	18. Q

EXERCISE 10-2

1. c	5. d	8. a
2. a	6. c	9. b
3. c	7. c	10. c
4. c		

EXERCISE 10-3

1. a	3. b	5. c
2. a	4. b	6. d

Chapter 11

EXERCISE 11-1

1. C	5. D	8. G
2. A	6. F	9. J
3. B	7. H	10. I
4. E		

EXERCISE 11-2

1. True	5. False	8. True
2. True	6. True	9. True
3. True	7. True	10. True
4. False		

EXERCISE 11-3

1. b	4. a	7. b
2. a	5. a	8. d
3. c	6. b	

Chapter 12

EXERCISE 12-1

1. I	5. B	8. F
2. J	6. C	9. G
3. A	7. D	10. H
4. E		

EXERCISE 12-2

1. True	5. False	8. True
2. True	6. True	9. True
3. True	7. False	10. False
4. True		

EXERCISE 12-3

1. d	5. c	8. c
2. b	6. d	9. d
3. c	7. b	10. a
4. d		

Chapter 13

EXERCISE 13-1

1. G	4. H	7. C
2. A	5. B	8. F
3. D	6. E	

EXERCISE 13-2

1. True	7. True	13. False
2. True	8. False	14. True
3. True	9. True	15. True
4. True	10. True	16. True
5. False	11. True	
6. False	12. True	

EXERCISE 13-3

1. d	4. d	6. c
2. a	5. d	7. b
3. d		

Chapter 14

EXERCISE 14-1

1. B	4. D	7. H
2. C	5. A	8. G
3. E	6. F	

EXERCISE 14-2

1. False	5. True	8. False
2. True	6. True	9. True
3. True	7. True	10. True
4. False		

EXERCISE 14-3

1. d	5. b	8. d
2. a	6. d	9. d
3. d	7. a	10. b
4. c		

Chapter 15

EXERCISE 15-1

1. B	4. D	7. F
2. C	5. E	8. I
3. A	6. G	9. H

EXERCISE 15-2

1. True	4. True	7. True
2. True	5. False	8. True
3. True	6. True	9. True

EXERCISE 15-3

1. a	5. d	8. d
2. c	6. d	9. c
3. d	7. c	10. a
4. c		

Chapter 16

EXERCISE 16-1

1. A	2. C	3. B

EXERCISE 16-2

1. Both refer to the seemingly elusive experience in which all things "click" and the person is free to respond at the highest level. A state of consciousness in which one becomes totally absorbed in what one is doing to the exclusion of all other thoughts and emotions.

2. Some appropriate questions to reveal how the client reached that state of being could be one of the most important challenges for the athlete on a given day. Simple, yet challenging questions can be framed as follows:
   - Can you tell me a time when you were on the field (or court etc.) and you were performing at your highest level?
   - Can you think of a time when it all came together for you?
   - What do you remember?
   - What were your thoughts?
   - What were you doing?
   - What were you aware of that allowed you to perform at that level?
   - What did you do to perform at your highest level?

3. A present focus on the task at hand has been referred to as a key ingredient in optimal performance. Questions that guide the athlete toward the present moment, toward activities that the athlete is in control of, and toward harnessing the key ingredients of the optimal mindset can assist in eliminating or reducing mental obstacles, emotional obstacles, or both.

EXERCISE 16-3

1. True	5. False	8. True
2. True	6. False	9. True
3. True	7. True	10. True
4. True		